The Globe's Best Diet

The Globe's Best Diet

Raymond Adamcik, MD

Raymond Adamcik, MD
DrAdamcik.com
GlobesBestDiet.com

iUniverse, Inc.
New York   Bloomington

The Globe's Best Diet
The Metabolic Syndrome Cure

The information, ideas, and suggestions in this book are not intended as a substitute for professional medical advice. Before following any suggestions contained in this book, you should consult your personal physician. Neither the author nor the publisher shall be liable or responsible for any loss or damage allegedly arising as a consequence of your use or application of any information or suggestions in this book.

iUniverse books may be ordered through booksellers or by contacting:

iUniverse
1663 Liberty Drive
Bloomington, IN 47403
www.iuniverse.com
1-800-Authors (1-800-288-4677)

Because of the dynamic nature of the Internet, any Web addresses or links contained in this book may have changed since publication and may no longer be valid. The views expressed in this work are solely those of the author and do not necessarily reflect the views of the publisher, and the publisher hereby disclaims any responsibility for them.

ISBN: 978-1-4401-2192-0 (pbk)
ISBN: 978-1-4401-2194-4 (cloth)
ISBN: 978-1-4401-2193-7 (ebk)

Printed in the United States of America

iUniverse rev. date: 2/13/2009

Contents

Introduction vii

Chapter 1: The Quick Fix 1

Chapter 2: The History of the Human Diet 6

Chapter 3: The Epidemic 12

Chapter 4: Healthy Motivation 17

Chapter 5: Cardio-Metabolic Syndrome 27

Chapter 6: Affecting Change. 33

Chapter 7: Irreplaceable Exercise. 37

Chapter 8: Relearning How—and What—to Eat 53

Chapter 9: Carbohydrates Simplified. 58

Chapter 10: Introducing the Villain—Insulin 69

Chapter 11: Momma and Popeye Were Right 73

Chapter 12: An Apple a Day is Bad for Business. 78

Chapter 13: The "Fats" of Life 81

Chapter 14: Amazing Omega-3 Fats—The Hidden Miracle . 83

Chapter 15: Nuts—the Secret Weight-Loss Weapon. 89

Chapter 16: Cooking and Salad Oils. 92

Chapter 17: Hidden Poisons in Your Diet and the
Trans-Fatty Acid Lies 95

Chapter 18: Saturated Fats. 101

Chapter 19: The New Hero—Flavonoids 107

Chapter 20: Alcohol—the Two-Faced Friend 112

Chapter 21: The Egg—Innocent or Guilty? 116

Chapter 22: Alternative Treatments 119

Chapter 23: Sample Diet 121

Conclusion. 125
Recipes. 127
Bibliography 145
About the Author 171
Acknowledgments 173
Index. 175

Introduction

As a practicing physician, I have spent the last thirty years in the trenches, counseling my patients about diet. I have devoted a lifetime to studying the subject while witnessing the explosion of obesity and diabetes in my practice, on the streets of America, and in my world travels. I have seen my patients struggle for a solution—many of them desperate, jumping into irrational and dangerous fad diets because of claims of short-term success, without any forethought as to the consequences and long-term effects on their health.

The study of diet has been my lifelong passion. I have read every diet book and scientific study that I could, hundreds in all—and for all the wrong and worthless information available, there has also been some good scientific research in this area, though the results are under-publicized. I have combined those findings with my knowledge of diets of the world and practical experience in the office, and have come to some conclusions: there are ways to control weight that are not only effective, but are also safe and healthy. These diets can reduce weight while greatly decreasing your chances of developing serious illnesses, such as coronary heart disease, diabetes, and cancer, and increasing your energy and vitality. Not only will you be slimmer, but you'll also live longer and feel better.

I know that many people will read *The Globe's Best Diet* as part of their search for the "holy grail" solution to obesity. But this diet is much more than an obesity treatment—it is a prescription for good health and life. Adopting this diet could save the lives of those who already suffer from diabetes, hypertension, cardio-metabolic syndrome, or coronary artery disease. Please share it with loved ones who suffer.

The Globe's Best Diet, which I am prescribing, is practical for every day and as a lifestyle. In fact, I have been living it myself since 2000.

At that time, I was on the verge of developing cardio-metabolic syndrome, which was a shock because I had been following the prescribed American Heart Association (AHA) diet perfectly. When it came to eating low-fat foods, I was the king—*and* I exercised regularly. How could my health not be perfect if my lifestyle was? Had I failed, or did the diet fail? I had to question the way I was living and everything that I had been taught.

After some desperate measures, I finally hit upon the Globe's Best Diet and found that I was able to lose weight and reverse my condition. I was actually able to *cure my cardio-metabolic syndrome!*

So I shared my secret with other doctors and patients, who were also amazed with their dramatic results. It shouldn't be surprising, though. Many populations of the world that adhere to the lifestyles in this book have unmatched health results.

The diet is not an untested fad. It is a return to our natural way of eating, nothing artificially altered or chemically processed— and I've included many fabulous recipes to help you start this simple and flavorful way of life.

In fact, your favorite part about the Globe's Best Diet may be the wonderful, natural food that you actually get to eat. But the *best* part about it will be the positive changes it has on your health and on every aspect of your life. Eat better, feel better, look better and live better through a better diet and lifestyle.

That's what I call a complete way of living!

Chapter 1: The Quick Fix

Everyone has a solution for weight problems. Just ask any overweight person on the street and they will be happy to share with you the "holy grail" solution they have found. But if their solution was so effective, it would be working for them! Opinions on this subject are like belly buttons—everybody has one. The number of fad diets is endless, and some are even comical: the grapefruit diet, the soup diet, the cabbage soup diet, the three-day diet, and, more recently, the wine-only diet. There are even familiar ones that seem more respectable, like the Atkins diet or the South Beach diet. But the reason there are so many diets and suggestions is that most of them fail.

Diet Don'ts
As a doctor, I have a problem with all of these diets. The body requires certain proteins, vitamins, minerals, and fats: altogether there are forty-five essential nutrients necessary for a healthy life. Many diets not only restrict calories but also severely restrict the types of food you can eat, therefore depriving your body of its essential nutrition. Basically, you can become malnourished, which may seem appealing from a caloric standpoint, but not when you consider what it does to your system. Sure, it seems somewhat ironic that obese people can be malnourished in our society, but it is entirely true.

Charging blindly into restrictive fad diets leaves many people deficient in essential nourishment—and there are myriad ways the body can react to this deficiency. You can become physically ill from a lack of vitamins, which is actually quite common. Vitamin D deficiency is rampant in the United States. Vitamin B deficiencies are common in the finicky elderly. Vitamin C deficiency can develop in the Atkins fanatic. There have even been deaths resulting among people who followed these fads.

If you leave out *any* of the forty-five essential nutrients, a deficiency will eventually manifest itself in some way—and a fad diet is sure to restrict your body's necessary nourishment. However, the possibility of physical harm is neither considered by the many nonmedical people who write fad diet books, nor is it considered by desperate, overweight people who are grasping for a quick fix. For most, short-term results are what count, not long-term negative health effects. And for that reason, they get what they want: a short-term weight loss only. But that soon fades into lifelong consequences.

What are the long-term effects of these fad diets? For the large part, they are unknown because the diets are so short lived. There have, however, been extensive studies on some long-term conditions that develop as a result of *not* getting the essential nutrients—and continued deficiencies can sometimes lead to death.

Protein deficiency, for example, can occur fairly easily in calorie-restricted diets if there is not significant food variety. A person who tries to lose weight by eating a high-carbohydrate diet low in fat and protein has the perfect setup for protein deficiency. People who limit themselves to just a few quirky foods can also become protein deficient, as can those on a starvation diet of six hundred calories or less.

What are the long-term effects of protein deficiency? If the food intake lacks sufficient calories or if the diet does not contain certain essential protein building blocks, then the body starts to use whatever it has around to spare. Optimistically, this would be fat and sugar stores. But if the body doesn't receive enough protein, it will start to break down its own muscle to get it.

Most people want to lose fat weight, not muscle. However,

2

it is hard to know which you are losing. If you get on the scale and the number is lower, you're happy. But what have you lost: fat or muscle mass? The answer can make a huge difference in your health.

Obviously, if you start to lose muscle, you could begin to feel physically weaker—although the long-term effects are much more serious than that. Muscle is the fastest metabolically active organ in the body. It is the engine that burns off the most calories in your system. Every time you lose muscle, your metabolic rate slows and your weight loss slows. Are you one of those people who go up and down in weight? Have you noticed that it gets harder to lose the weight each time? This is because you have been starving away muscle.

Every time you lose weight, you preserve less muscle and your metabolism is slower for the next attempted weight loss. Diets that are deficient in protein are doomed to failure. Not only won't they work, they will actually aggravate the problem by promoting weight gain once regular intake is resumed but metabolic rate is still low.

In other words, if you lose weight on a diet that is severely restricted in calories or protein, your short-term smile will be replaced by lifelong problems with obesity. The result you achieve will be the exact opposite of your goal.

In fact, *all* of the fad diets are doomed to failure. That's why "diet" is just another four-letter word. Everybody wants the quick cure, the magic pill you take to wake up a hundred pounds lighter. Quit dreaming! Weight gain is a process that develops over many years of a faulty lifestyle, so it is unrealistic to expect to solve this problem with a brief and drastic change. What you need is not a new diet, but a new lifestyle.

Living for the Long Term

Most dieters are on a sprint. We doctors hear it all the time: "I lost thirty pounds my first month!" But how much weight do they gain back the second month? In six months? The likely answer is: "All of it and more." There is also a good chance that, in the process, they have lost muscle, in this way permanently slowing the body's metabolism. And they may have also robbed themselves of essential nutrients. What these dieters are doing is attempting a large chemistry experiment on their bodies. In most cases, the experiment fails and they become the victims.

The number one problem with most diets is that they try to cure a lifetime of bad lifestyle habits with a short-term treatment. Once you stop that treatment and return to your old lifestyle, your weight will return to its former setting—only now, you may have lost some of your muscle mass, too. With a lower metabolic rate, you are sure to put on even more weight. This goes to show that *you cannot cure a lifelong problem with a short-term solution!* You may even make matters worse.

The second problem with these diets is people's expectations. Everyone would like to lose *all* of that extra weight and keep it off. Realistically, only a tiny percentage can succeed in huge weight loss. You have to set a realistic goal for yourself that will be achievable by making and maintaining certain lifestyle changes. That goal should be about 10 percent of your body weight, at most. If you weigh 300 pounds and can get down to 270 and maintain that, then it is a realistic, sustainable goal. You will also see many benefits in terms of health, appearance, and general well-being when you achieve that weight loss of 10 percent. If you strive for the moon (or your high school pants size) too quickly, however, you will become frustrated halfway to your goal and give up, returning to where you started—or worse.

Sure, there are some people who lose beyond 10 percent of their body weight and keep it off, but it is really quite rare. To accomplish this takes exceptional changes in lifestyle. It also requires a highly motivated individual who must maintain strict discipline—and most people would not have weight problems to begin with if they were that disciplined!

For those who think they may fit into the highly disciplined category, I will tell you what your best chances to accomplish drastic weight loss are later in the book. For now, however, I recommend that most people think about setting a realistic goal—and *The Globe's Best Diet* will help you get there.

This program was developed after a lifetime of extensive research into published studies of dietary modifications. I have personally been the guinea pig for some of these findings, and have used these recommendations with over three thousand of my own patients through twenty-five years of medical practice. The lifestyle I am prescribing is highly effective in promoting weight loss in a safe, healthy, and sustainable manner—otherwise, as a medical professional, I wouldn't be suggesting it.

Until now, my research was only available through an office visit. However, I have decided to share my passion for this subject with millions of readers in the knowledge that I could help them … if only I could reach them.

The weight loss goals I'll help you set and achieve will be realistic—but the effects on your life will be truly unbelievable!

Chapter 2: The History of the Human Diet

Why learn history? It is said that those who do not learn from the past are destined to repeat it. This may be especially true for dieters.

I want you to understand where some of society's misconceptions about diet started—and there is a lot of misinformation out there! Worse yet, you have been lied to, and these lies have become so ingrained in our society that they are commonly believed to be true. Once we dispel the myths and misinformation, you will be able to make better decisions about your own diet.

So Simple, Even a Caveman Could Diet!

Man has had half a million years' experience with diet. In caveman days, there were no dieticians or physicians; they survived in spite of their total ignorance of nutritional requirements or recommendations. Cavemen could not go to the local convenience store or be lured by the "golden arches." Somehow, they managed quite well without counting fats and carbohydrates or by following the American Heart Association guidelines.

Early humans survived on whatever they could forage for approximately a hundred thousand generations. They were predominantly hunters and gatherers and lived off what the earth provided naturally.

The caveman diet was rich in a large number of plants, and the meat intake mostly consisted of game foods. The herding of animals had not yet been achieved, so game was hunted intensely—and animals are lower in fat and higher in protein in a wild state. Early humans' activity level was naturally very high. Food was not readily available in the immediate vicinity, so hunting and gathering trips were required to provide for basic necessities. On these excursions, they picked fresh fruit, vegetables, and nuts of all different varieties and color. They knew that those things tasted good. But we now know that multicolored skins contain flavonoids, naturally occurring chemicals that protect us against certain diseases (which we will discuss in more detail later). There was no processing of carbohydrate-rich foods, and items such as white bread, pasta, processed candies, and cereals, which modern humans seem to think we can't live without, were unimaginable back then. If sugars were available at all, they were eaten in their natural state.

A typical food pyramid currently has at its base six servings of bread, cereals, pasta, and rice. (Figure 1)

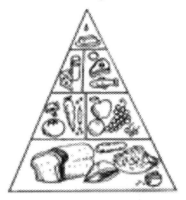

Figure 1 AHA Food Pyramid

According to the USDA and AHA, these foods are recommended as the mainstay of our diet, outnumbering all the other food groups. A caveman couldn't find these carb-heavy foods, yet he survived for hundreds of thousands of years without them in any significant quantity. How, then, have they become considered such a big part of our "essential" daily nutrition?

The AHA would have you eating 55 percent of your diet in carbohydrates alone, with cookies, cakes, and oils in the top tier. A caveman most likely would not have enjoyed this pyramid, preferring a handful of cherries to a stalk of wheat any day.

The Effects of Agriculture and Industry

What happened is that around five hundred generations ago, some populations began developing agriculture. Initially, they focused on the easiest things to grow, such as rice and wheat. However, these harvests were very labor intensive: planting, reaping, grinding, and cooking were all done manually. There was no processing or removal of fiber or other nutrients, so the harvests consisted of whole-grain products. Since a fair amount of physical exercise was required just to be able to eat these carbohydrate-rich crops, they were consumed sparingly.

Only the last ten generations have benefited from the Industrial Revolution. Machines now do much of our labor for us: tractors plow fields and harvesters reap them. The amount of physical exertion needed to produce a carb-heavy meal has been drastically reduced—and we can see the effects it has had on our waistlines.

So far, only the last two or three generations have survived the current processed food era. Foods naturally rich in fiber and nutrients are sent to factories, where they are ground down, the healthy fibers are removed, and the essential nutrients, like vitamins, flavonoids, and minerals, are lost. This is all done without human physical labor. Then these products are transported to your local convenience store or supermarket, where people drive to buy this cheap, processed, high-carbohydrate, low-nutrition "food." Is it any wonder that obesity is now rampant in our society? We are experiencing an "experimental" diet now that has never in history been higher in effortless, sugary foods.

The AHA condones this diet full of carbohydrate-rich foods

as "healthy," even though there is no evidence to show what long-term effects it will have on us as a whole. How could there be if such a diet has never existed before in human history? We are in the midst of a massive experiment to see what will occur when we continue to push huge amounts of carbohydrate-rich foods on world populations. Let's just say that the early results have not been favorable.

Longer Lives, Lower Quality of Living

Up until this processed food era, medicine was in its infancy. Its prior focus was the treatment of infectious diseases that were usually fatal by the age of forty. Much of the population didn't live to experience the complications of poor diet; in fact, a little extra weight was helpful to stave off illness. Most people lived on farms, where they ate a variety of natural foods and their activity level was very high. Any carbohydrates they consumed were burned off through physical labor.

In 1945, the age of antibiotics started to extend life expectancy. As people began to live longer, heart attacks emerged as the number one killer in our society, and a landmark seven-country study was undertaken to determine the possible reasons. Populations affected most were those in northern climate countries, like America and Finland; countries with warmer climates, such as those along the Mediterranean, seemed to be spared from this epidemic.

The difference in the rate of coronary disease among different countries was dramatic, with occurrences seventeen times greater in some populations than in others. The rate in the United States was four times that of Greece, particularly the island of Crete. The study examined various factors and found that diet played the biggest role in determining the cases of heart disease within a country. Based on these results, dietary recommendations were made, with the main message being: "Follow a low-fat diet."

Americans, who are generally good patients, listened. But in the process, new diseases were born. It turned out that the correct message had not been delivered, and there were obvious flaws in the low-fat theory.

For one, Eskimos had superb protection from heart problems, even with their diet high in fat, which is almost exclusively derived from fish. The French seemed immune to heart disease, too, in spite of their butter-rich diet, and this inconsistency has come to be known as "the French paradox." Interestingly, even the diet in Greece was not low-fat; it was extremely high in olive oil usage, but there was very little beef intake. There was also the Japanese case to consider, where the population was protected from heart disease in spite of a high smoking rate. Their diet was not low-fat, either, but was rich in soybeans, fish, and tea. It was clear that the low-fat answer could not explain all of these inconsistencies.

Dueling Diets

Around the time that these cracks in the theory were being called into question, we heard another voice, that of Dr. Robert Atkins, who shouted an opposing message: "Eat a low-carbohydrate, high-fat and protein diet." It was heresy to the medical profession, but individuals gave testimony to its effectiveness. Patients loved it because they saw results—and they were allowed to go back to the beef that had been forbidden to them on the low-fat diet.

Still, the medical profession's low-fat concept had a steady number of adherents, some of whom even took it one step further: if low-fat is good, really low-fat must be better. Thus, the Pritikin and Ornish diets were born, increasing the recommended carbohydrate intake from 55 percent to between 80 and 90 percent. Patients tried to comply, but a diet of cardboard was tough to follow. The few who did stick to it were experimenting with yet another untested diet since there were no healthy countries that exclusively ate carbohydrate-rich foods. It was based on an incorrect premise to begin with. Low-fat was not the answer, so really low-fat was worse.

That's when some good ideas turned into disasters. Further

review of the seven-country study brought forth the idea that vegetable fat was okay but dairy and animal fats were the main culprits. That concept is actually correct, but what sprung from it is responsible for many deaths around the world. In an attempt to minimize dairy and beef fat, a new poison was entered into the global diet: the trans-fatty acid.

Vegetable fat, like olive oil, is a healthy liquid, which made it inconvenient for packaging and spreading. Consumers wanted something more solid, like butter. It was discovered that if a vegetable fat were modified, it could be made more solid (a good example is margarine). This poisonous concoction spread worldwide with incredible speed and was touted as a healthy substitute to those bad animal and dairy fats. As people tried hard to eat this foul stuff, they became progressively sicker. There was no scientific proof that these chemicals were safe or healthy, yet they were distributed like candy across the globe, bringing us further from a healthy solution.

So, what does this historical overview mean? Which diet is right? Where did we go wrong? What is a person to do on a day-to-day basis? Who can you believe, and how can you combat the obesity and health issues that have emerged from this path of dietary destruction?

The answers are contained in these chapters.

Chapter 3: The Epidemic

Are your clothes fitting tighter these days? Has your weight been creeping up year after year? Do you have more than one wardrobe to accommodate each size you have been? If your answer is yes to any of these questions, then you are part of the epidemic.

"Which epidemic?" you're probably wondering. "Isn't that like a flu that hits a bunch of people all of a sudden?"

No, this one is even more insidious. It is the obesity epidemic, and it has been sneaking up on the American and worldwide public for thirty or forty years, bringing with it an epidemic of all the illnesses associated with obesity.

Americans were the first affected by this epidemic, and they were hit hard. Our Western diet was predominantly to blame, but recently the rest of the world is rapidly following. Our culture, particularly our poor diet habits, has been spreading everywhere.

The bad news is that this epidemic is just as dangerous as infectious ones like pneumonia and the flu. In fact, it is even deadlier. Weight gain is now overtaking smoking as the number-one killer. It is estimated that 64.5 percent of Americans are overweight, 30.5 percent fit the classification of obese, and 5 percent are severely obese.

Obesity skyrocketed between 1960 and 2000. Among men, it went from 11 to 28 percent, and from 16 to 34 percent among women. These trends were even worse in some subgroups. African American women and Hispanics now had an overweight prevalence in the 60 to 80 percent range and obesity rates approach 50 percent. Medicine had been successfully extending our lifespan during these decades, but the trend will soon reverse to shorter life expectancy due to this obesity epidemic.

The Spread of a Deadly Disease

How did we get ourselves in such a mess? There are many reasons. In America, we are very fortunate to live in a land of plenty. Agriculture and the food industry have gone high-tech, and machines work very inexpensively with minimal human labor. This makes for plentiful and cheap food.

In many countries, fields are still plowed by hand or with the assistance of beasts of burden. But here, expensive agricultural equipment minimizes physical labor for humans. A combine can harvest enough wheat in eight seconds to make seventy-three loaves of bread. These mechanically grown and harvested foods are then reprocessed by the food industry, which contributes greatly to the epidemic.

I've already mentioned that during processing fiber, vitamins, and essential nutrients are removed. But what I didn't tell you is that after the foods are reprocessed, they are more concentrated in calories than they were in their original state. Carbohydrates that are naturally present in grains are no longer bound to fibers but are reduced to pure sugars.

Sure, who doesn't like sweet-tasting food? After all, it is what we Americans are accustomed to. But these foods are not natural. They are vitamin deficient, energy –rich, and nutrition poor. They are a pale substitute for actual, essential food.

This reprocessed material is mechanically packaged and boxed, and magically appears at your grocer, local convenience store, or in a vending machine in the company break room. So, we have lots of cheap choices because of technology, but the food itself is lacking in nutrition and packed with calories.

There is another problem with this processed food, since it is often chemically altered. A harmful additive called trans-fatty acid is commonly introduced during processing. Although this in itself doesn't have any specific effect on obesity, it will certainly have harmful consequences for the body in several ways, which we will discuss later.

Another cause of the epidemic besides cheap, bad food is changing lifestyles. And the worst among these is decreased physical activity. For some people, switching on the PlayStation is the closest they care to come to exercise. But physical activity doesn't have to be as painful as you may think.

In other countries, there is no lack of exercise; there is what they call "work." Many jobs in different parts of the world require extreme physical activity. Farming is a good example; before the Industrial Revolution, the majority of the world's population was employed as farmers. In some areas today, especially third-world countries, this remains the case.

Many other forms of employment also demand more activity in other regions. Take, for instance, the construction business. Here caterpillars, cranes, jackhammers, nail guns, etc. are labor-saving devices that have replaced massive amounts of human physical activity. In other countries, they are nonexistent. Furthermore, most Americans are employed in service positions that involve deskwork and decreased physical activity.

So, Americans sit for a living and eat calorie-rich junk. Is that all? Unfortunately, no, there is more. Consider how we get to work, to our friends' houses or to the corner store. In Europe, where gas and autos are too expensive for many, they walk. But walking has almost completely disappeared from our society. We are in such a rush that we drive to the local convenience store only a block away. It is not unusual for Europeans to walk several miles to a store, but in America this would be highly atypical— almost unthinkable.

Sometimes, Americans will go to extremes just to avoid burning off a little energy. I have seen people jump in the car to literally go down the block a few houses or get on the elevator to go up a floor. In short, we have become lazy. Saving time has become top priority to most people, even over maintaining their health.

Worse yet, our children's lack of activity has extended far beyond our own. Obesity has recently tripled in children between the ages of two and five, and has also tripled since 1970 for those between six and nineteen years old. Abdominal obesity in particular has increased 65 to 70 percent among the younger population. This explosion of obesity in our youth will cause heart disease to triple by the time this generation hits fifty! That is not the future we want for our kids.

When I was a child, I was always outside with my friends, playing sports and partaking in physical exercise. Now, videogames, cable TV, and DVDs make home a far more popular place than the local park.

So, we have cheap, calorie-rich, nutritionally-poor food that is tainted with poisons; we have stopped most physical work; we use cars to avoid any possible chance of exercise; and we are distracted by electronic entertainment—all traits we are passing on to our children. There can't possibly be more to this epidemic … yet there is.

Advice from "Dear Flabby"

Lastly, we have been given bad advice. The medical profession has been saying for the last thirty years that the low-fat diet is the healthiest. It was thought to lower cholesterol and therefore lower the risk of heart disease, which is what that seven-country study was all about.

It was also believed that a low-fat diet aided in weight loss. The logic went like this: Fat is very calorie-intense; there are nine calories in one gram of fat. But there are only four calories in one gram of carbohydrate or protein. So, if you cut out the item highest in calories (fat), you should naturally lose weight.

Based on that equation, the low-fat diet has been recommended for weight loss by the medical profession since I graduated from medical school in 1978. Throughout twenty-two years of practice, I had repeated the mantra that I had heard over and over again: patients will lose weight by following a low-fat diet, which is healthy and good for your heart. Even now, a large portion of the medical field continues to endorse this theory.

There was a problem, though. My patients weren't losing weight.

Of course, I had a good explanation for that: they must be doing it wrong! They were cheating or not exercising—*they* had to be at fault somehow. Some of them even started to gain weight on this diet. The audacity of them!

It took me many years to understand why, but my period of enlightenment began when I realized that it was the mantra that was wrong! A low-fat diet will make you fat! It was all a hoax.

So, we finally seem to have our answer: we eat malnourishing food; don't exercise at, after, to, or from work; enjoy slouching on our couches; and have been following the wrong diet because of bad advice that has been passed along from the medical profession for decades. Hence, an epidemic of bad lifestyle habits has promoted an epidemic of medical illness. Now you understand how we got into this twenty-first century dilemma.

The question is: How do we get out of it?

Chapter 4: Healthy Motivation

Most people look at the whole idea of weight gain with an apathetic attitude. They accept it as a part of getting older or leading a busy lifestyle. It's popular—everyone is doing it!

There are social aspects to being fat. Recent studies show that if you hang around with an overweight crowd, you are more likely to accept the idea and develop a similar lifestyle and appearance. You can actually *catch* obesity.

Many individuals think of weight gain only from a cosmetic perspective. They know it is considered unattractive and suggests to others that they are not physically fit. It says that they don't care enough about themselves to take care of themselves and is a statement of low self-worth.

The problem is that most people aren't aware of the longer-term effects of slow weight gain. First, a few pounds are overlooked, then a few more and a few more. Each of these steps increases harm to the body, and eventually very serious consequences result.

What are they? We all know the basics: it's bad for your heart and you can get diabetes if you gain enough weight. But this is really only scratching the surface of what weight can do to your health—and how it can shorten your life.

Many of the consequences of obesity are only now being defined. A good example of a relatively new illness is cardio-metabolic syndrome. This was not even a known condition when I was in medical school; now we recognize that it affects millions. The cardio-metabolic syndrome is a cluster of conditions that cumulatively damage the cardiovascular system and leads to increased risk of obesity-related diseases like hearts attack, stroke, diabetes, and death. The cardio-metabolic syndrome will be discussed extensively in chapter five. It has always been present, but medical science was unaware of its serious health implications. Since obesity has exploded, cardio-metabolic syndrome has skyrocketed.

It is my hope that if people are more aware of such risks resulting from their behavior, they will be more motivated to make changes. In the following paragraphs, many readers will be able to identify symptoms they already have or are in the process of developing. Don't look away. It is my hope and purpose to spur you on and motivate you to make the essential lifestyle choices you need in order to reverse these conditions. Now is the time to go beyond the basics.

Recognizing the Risks

We all know that weight gain looks bad, but what else are you getting yourself into? What will your future look like? And what are the effects of this epidemic? Well, there are many—all of them bad.

In the earlier phases of weight gain, there may be no obvious symptoms. Most Americans start gaining about two to five pounds a year starting in their twenties—though, as I have stated, this problem is showing up even earlier as our lifestyles have worsened. Most of my patients use the ostrich approach regarding this weight creep: they refuse to get on a scale. What they don't see doesn't exist. We call this ***denial***.

You have to overcome denial and accept that you are developing a problem in order to have any chance of modifying it. Even small amounts of weight gain can have an effect over time. Studies show that people who maintain the weight they had at a younger age (say, twenty-five) experience significant health benefits when they reach fifty. So those few pounds that you put on each year that you accept as normal can have dramatic effects on how you feel and act at the still-youngish age of fifty.

At a rate of twenty to thirty pounds a decade, many middle-aged people will be at least fifty pounds overweight. They will have far less physical function, and their activity levels will suffer. Can you imagine carrying around a fifty-pound weight everywhere you go? I would certainly jump in my car to see a neighbor if I had that heavy dumbbell to bring with me.

Even people who limit their weight gain to ten to thirty pounds during the ensuing decades are far less active than those who manage to keep it to ten pounds or less. Individuals who aren't able to stay within ten pounds of their weight at age twenty-five feel the pain, too. They ache significantly more, and the extra pounds start to have a wear and tear effect on the weight-bearing joints of the knees, hips, and back; every step will put extra pressure on those joints and, eventually, they start to deteriorate. These people will also enter the early phases of arthritis at fifty.

Those unable to stay close to their weight at age twenty-five have less vitality, energy, and vigor as well. Not only will they not maintain their activity levels, they really just won't even feel like doing much anymore. Their life will already start being progressively limited. They will continue living in a smaller and smaller box, awaiting their final box.

In addition, weight gainers feel worse emotionally. Some of this may just be the metabolic effects of bad food. Those pollutants circulate into your brain, slowing you down both mentally and physically, and you just don't feel too well. That's why depression in obese people is pretty common.

Besides these initial effects on the mind and body, you are already in the process of developing a lethal disease. Those who have gained thirty pounds or more between the ages of twenty-five and fifty are already significantly at risk of DYING FROM THEIR WEIGHT GAIN. An increase of that amount also increases the risk of death 53 percent more than those who have managed to maintain their weight during the years. That's close to being a smoker, for which the risk of death is thought to be about 60 percent higher than for nonsmokers. You are literally taking your life into your hands.

The Numbers Don't Lie

Most people think of a slow thirty-pound weight gain as a minor problem or annoyance. They point to the guy next to them who has gained fifty or more pounds. Okay, so he's sick, too. It doesn't make *your* condition any better.

Wake up, all you round-in-the-middle people! You are part of a crisis situation, and your life is already on the line. It is time for action and to get back on track. You need to regain your physical activity to look and feel better. You must stop your senseless crawl into the smaller and smaller boxes and reclaim your vitality and your life. How? By changing your lifestyle.

Some people truly don't know where they stand in all of this. Are you almost normal, overweight, obese, or severely obese? Do you know? Most people want to underestimate this. "I am full-figured." "I have love handles." Are those really just nice ways of saying "obese"? Here is how you can find out definitively.

The Body Mass Indicator (BMI) is a standard medical tool used to determine the level of obesity present. It can be easily calculated based on standard height and weight measurements.

First you need to know your height in inches and your weight in pounds. Then consult the table below to determine your BMI.. (Table 1).

Start with your height in inches, then follow the row sideways until you reach your weight. Then follow that column to the top row to get your BMI. For example; if your height is 61 inches, and your weight is 158, your BMI would be 31.

Table 1 BMI Table

BMI	19	20	21	22	23	24	25	26	27	28	29	30	31	32	33	34	35
Height (inches)								Body Weight (pounds)									
58	91	96	100	105	110	115	119	124	129	134	138	143	148	153	158	162	167
59	94	99	104	109	114	119	124	128	133	138	143	148	153	158	163	168	173
60	97	102	107	112	118	123	128	133	138	143	148	153	158	163	168	174	179
61	100	106	111	116	122	127	132	137	143	148	153	158	164	169	174	180	185
62	104	109	115	120	126	131	136	142	147	153	158	164	169	175	180	186	191
63	107	113	118	124	130	135	141	146	152	158	163	169	175	180	186	191	197
64	110	116	122	128	134	140	145	151	157	163	169	174	180	186	192	197	204
65	114	120	126	132	138	144	150	156	162	168	174	180	186	192	198	204	210
66	118	124	130	136	142	148	155	161	167	173	179	186	192	198	204	210	216
67	121	127	134	140	146	153	159	166	172	178	185	191	198	204	211	217	223
68	125	131	138	144	151	158	164	171	177	184	190	197	203	210	216	223	230
69	128	135	142	149	155	162	169	176	182	189	196	203	209	216	223	230	236
70	132	139	146	153	160	167	174	181	188	195	202	209	216	222	229	236	243
71	136	143	150	157	165	172	179	186	193	200	208	215	222	229	236	243	250
72	140	147	154	162	169	177	184	191	199	206	213	221	228	235	242	250	258
73	144	151	159	166	174	182	189	197	204	212	219	227	235	242	250	257	265
74	148	155	163	171	179	186	194	202	210	218	225	233	241	249	256	264	272
75	152	160	168	176	184	192	200	208	216	224	232	240	248	256	264	272	279
76	156	164	172	180	189	197	205	213	221	230	238	246	254	263	271	279	287

If your BMI is less than 18.5, you are underweight. If it is between 18.5 and 25, your weight is normal for your height. If your BMI is 25 to 30, you are classified as overweight. If it is 30 to 40, you are obese. If your BMI is over 40, you fall into the category of severely obese.

That should give you a general measure as to how serious your problem is. Health issues start increasing with a BMI above 25—but the time to start a better lifestyle is now, regardless of where you stand. If your BMI is 26 and you have bad lifestyle habits, you will progress into obesity before you know it.

How Weight Gain Affects Your Health and Threatens Your Life

Obesity affects multiple organ systems, the most obvious of which is the cardiovascular system. I think everyone looks at a really fat person and thinks to themselves that he probably has or is going to have a heart condition. What's the connection? For one thing, the more you weigh, the higher your blood pressure.

Blood pressure is directly correlated with weight; 80 percent of people who lose weight see a drop in their blood pressure. For every pound you lose, the upper number of your reading (systolic pressure) goes down two points, and the lower number (diastolic) goes down one. Even a five- to ten-pound weight loss can make a difference between whether or not you need to take daily medication to control your blood pressure.

One of the most dreaded and serious complications related to obesity is diabetes (diabetes mellitus). The fact is that it really doesn't take much weight gain to multiply your risk of this disease. Only eleven to eighteen extra pounds will double your chances of developing it, and that risk increases exponentially with additional weight gain. For example, a forty-pound weight gain is associated with a quadruple risk of developing diabetes.

If you are like most of my patients, you may respond apathetically to that risk. Most patients fear diabetes only because of the needles involved. If they don't have to face the needle then they are not too worried. However, I have a tremendous fear of that condition because of my medical experience.

There has been a complete explosion of diabetes in America, which is related to the factors I discussed in the previous chapter. When I first started my practice, I would see patients who were diabetic only occasionally. Now, they have come to dominate my appointments. When I began in medicine, the rate of diabetes was 4 percent in adults; currently, it has doubled to 8 percent.

I see diabetic patients about five times more frequently than I see other patients because they are at a very high risk of medical complications. Their chances of a heart attack and stroke go up seven times, and they are at increased risk of kidney failure, blindness, amputations, and early death. It is for all these reasons that I fear diabetes.

Our country is quickly becoming a land of diabetics, however. Many of you reading this book already suffer from it. But the Globe's Best Diet is a detour on the road toward diabetes, taking you in another, healthier direction altogether. I have successfully used this diet to prevent diabetes and to treat it effectively in many of my patients.

The problem, though, is even worse in children. Young people are marching rapidly down the road toward diabetes, following in the footsteps of their parents. Type II, or so-called adult diabetes, is now occurring ten times more frequently than it was in the past. In fact, due to weight gain, more kids are getting the adult form of Type II diabetes than Type I, the juvenile form. As Bob Dylan said, "The times they are a-changing."

Diabetes means death to your cardiovascular system. The blood vessels are destroyed at an extremely rapid rate and the atherosclerotic process is accelerated in the arteries, affecting the heart, brain, legs, and kidneys (in men it also causes impotency by affecting penile blood flow).

When the circulation to your extremities is affected, it can cause gangrene, resulting in amputations. The kidneys can be destroyed, resulting in dialysis. And the blood vessels in the eyes can be destroyed, resulting in adult blindness. Overall, the effects on the body are devastating and often fatal. That's why diabetes is on my top ten list of serious illnesses.

The good news is that lifestyle changes can protect you from this disease. Aggressive interventions can reduce your risk of developing diabetes by 58 percent. For those who already have diabetes, its complications can be prevented or kept to a minimum with lifestyle changes. In fact, with sustained weight loss, the condition can become dormant, and some people are able to bring their numbers back down to the normal range.

The bad news is that with obesity raising your risks of diabetes, high blood pressure, and heart disease, it's no wonder that other risks also multiply—like that of cancer. Yes, you greatly increase your risk of this deadly and dreaded disease by becoming obese. It's not so easy to ignore that slow weight gain now, is it?

There are eight types of cancer correlated with obesity: breast, uterus, cervix, colon, esophagus, pancreas, kidney, and prostrate. Obese patients have higher risks of developing all of these. So the next time you see an obese person (even if you're looking in the mirror), maybe you shouldn't be thinking about eventual heart disease. Instead, you may say to yourself, "I bet that person is at risk for cancer."

A Grocery List of Illnesses

If cancer isn't enough to get you to change your lifestyle, maybe a more complete list of other illnesses will. As fat accumulates in your body, some gets stored in your liver. This can start to inflame the organ, which, with time, can progress to cirrhosis (permanent scarring and liver failure). Most people think that only alcoholics get this condition, but obesity is another common cause.

Weight gain can bring about other complications as well, such as sleep apnea. As fat accumulates in the neck and throat, breathing passages can be blocked off during sleep. The result is snoring, and impaired and intermittently blocked breathing. On the lower side of the spectrum, you might wind up sleeping alone. But more serious implications include sleeplessness and progressive daytime fatigue, oxygen deficiency, and fatal heart irregularities that can occur during sleep. So this is yet another way that obesity can kill you.

But let's not forget about its other far-reaching effects, such as those on the gastrointestinal system. If you are one of the millions of people suffering from heartburn or gastro-esophageal reflux (GERD), it is likely that weight gain has been causing your symptoms. Overweight people have a double risk of this condition, and it triples in the obese. That pain is trying to tell you something, so listen to your body and make some changes.

Gallbladder attacks are more common in obese people and frequently result in hospitalization and surgical removal. With surgical intervention, this condition is usually not fatal, but painful, food-initiated attacks can go on for years.

Gout is another excruciating complication from weight gain. It occurs far more often in obese people with rich diets, causing sudden, extremely painful swelling of the joints. If you have ever had a gout attack, you will want to do anything to avoid another one—even adopt a healthier lifestyle.

Arthritis is an inevitable consequence of obesity. The stress of carrying around all those extra pounds puts tremendous pressure on the weight-bearing joints (particularly the hips, knees, and spine) and, of course, your feet suffer also. This develops into a catch-22 situation: in order to lose weight, these obese arthritics need to exercise, but because of pain and limited mobility, they cannot. This lack of exercise means that their only chance of weight loss comes from cutting down aggressively on their food intake, but even this is not very effective without physical activity. These people usually have pretty slow metabolic rates from years of improper dieting, so weight loss is difficult to maintain even with restricted calories. Eventually, these individuals gain more weight, the arthritis is aggravated by the extra pounds, and activity is limited even further. In such a situation, weight loss can become nearly impossible (though I will give you some hints about how to approach this later).

In women, obesity can wreak havoc on the hormonal and reproductive systems. The excess fat throws off the hormonal balance, resulting in irregular cycles and fertility problems. For men, it hits you where it really hurts: obesity is one of the major causes of impotence. There are a lot of things most men are willing to give up to sustain their lazy lifestyles, but sexual function is usually at the bottom of the list.

Obesity can also cause swelling of the lower extremities (edema), which can result in unsightly discolorations of the skin. Eventually ulcerations and infections follow, as well as more potentially serious complications such as phlebitis (blood clots). Obesity can even affect unlikely organs like the eye with an increased risk of cataract formations.

Had enough of the health problems? Well, the psychological and social effects of obesity can also be profound. Obese people often have bad issues with self-esteem, seeing themselves as unworthy or at fault. This lack of self-esteem can have dramatic repercussions on their work performance and social life.

Cosmetically, obese people appear significantly older than their slim counterparts, and there is a great deal of social prejudice against them. They are stereotyped as lazy and not in control of themselves; therefore, they are often not respected or desired by others.

Death by Chocolate (and Other Foods)

If this is still not enough to convince you to make the changes you need, there is always the risk of death. It is estimated that excess weight now accounts for 7.7 percent of premature deaths in men and 11.75 percent in women. The bottom line is that excess weight isn't just about looking fat. It can clearly be fatal.

You don't have to live this way. You don't have to die this way. These problems are largely related to poor lifestyle choices and can to some extent be protected against by something as simple as better quality food. You can change your lifestyle and become healthier; therefore, you can change the outcome of this deadly epidemic.

Make the decision to change your future—but start today.

Chapter 5: Cardio-Metabolic Syndrome

Before we move on to lifestyle changes, I want to highlight one last complication caused by weight gain. This condition is so serious and prevalent that it warrants a separate chapter. If you are reading this book because you are concerned about your weight, there is a fairly good chance that you already have cardio-metabolic syndrome and may not even know it!

Until 2006, cardio-metabolic syndrome was only called metabolic syndrome. In the more distant past it was known as syndrome X and was first described in 1988. Now we know it as cardio-metabolic syndrome because of the profound effects it has on the cardiovascular system.

I was pretty shocked when, in 2000, I found out that I was on the verge of developing this illness, which was an unknown condition when I was in medical school. Sure, it existed, but no one yet realized its risks and implications or recognized it as a distinct condition. At the time of the diagnosis, I was living what I thought was an ideal lifestyle, according to what I had been taught. I had been a regular exerciser since 1984, kept my weight in a fairly tight range, and had followed the prescribed low-fat diet religiously. In fact, I "improved" on what was recommended, which was to limit fat intake to 30 percent and eat a diet rich in carbohydrates.

For higher-risk patients, a more rigorous restriction of fat was advised, and for those with heart conditions, fat content was decreased to 20 or 25 percent. Some physicians carried the diet to the extreme. The Pritikin diet advocated limiting fat to 10 percent of one's daily intake; of the remaining calories, up to 90 percent were to be derived from carbohydrates.

It was considered medical wisdom at the time that the lower your fat intake, the healthier you were living. I was great at following my own advice and figured, why do it only halfway? I shot for a diet as low in fat as possible. It was large quantities of pasta or rice every night; chickens and cows applauded when I walked by. My diet was just about as low in fat as I could get without becoming a strict vegetarian.

Then I did a specialized blood test that looks at types of cholesterol and found out that my insides were about to explode! I flunked the blood test with flying colors. For one thing, my triglycerides were extremely elevated at 400. This number should be no more than 100–150. I also found out that my good cholesterol was extremely low at 29. It should be at least 40; for someone like me, an avid runner, it should be around 50 or more. For the heck of it, I also had my insulin level tested. It should be around 10, but mine was 40—in the diabetic range. My blood sugar was also borderline elevated at 105. It should be less than 100. What had gone wrong with my perfect lifestyle?

It was then that I renewed my research into diets and dietary history and discussed my findings with colleagues. My low-fat, high-carbohydrate diet had resulted in borderline cardio-metabolic syndrome.

After researching, I put myself on a drastically different diet and, several months later, had fantastic results. I had lost twenty pounds (which was all I needed to lose) and my blood tests were not only corrected to normal, but were even in the better-than-average range. I began to share my dietary experience with my patients, and many of them not only lost weight but were also able to reverse their cardio-metabolic syndrome.

How Do You Know if You Have It?

I began to research this newly coined diagnosis more extensively. In case you haven't heard, cardio-metabolic syndrome is considered the disease of the new millennium. About 25 percent of adults have it—and about forty-five million people in the United States suffer from it. This syndrome is so prevalent that it will contribute more to the development of heart disease than smoking.

So exactly what is it? Here are the criteria for diagnosis:

Waist circumference: Men > 41 inches, Women > 35 inches
Triglycerides: ≥ 150 mg/dl
HDL cholesterol: Men < 40 mg/dl, Women < 50mg/dl
Blood pressure: ≥ 130/85
Fasting blood sugar: ≥ 110

Of these five criteria, a showing of three or more is considered sufficient to make a positive diagnosis of cardio-metabolic syndrome.

Many of you reading this may not know your numbers for triglycerides, HDL cholesterol, blood pressure, or blood sugar, but I bet you have a pretty good idea what your waist size is. To me, the waist size is the most important criterion since the correlation among weight, waist size, and abnormalities in blood sugar, body lipids, and blood pressure is extremely strong.

However, if your waist size is less than indicated above, you are still not in the clear. Many people who have the syndrome have had less drastic changes in their waist sizes, but if you are twenty pounds or more heavier than your high school weight, consider yourself a candidate for this condition. Really, everybody—including you—should at some time be screened for cardio-metabolic syndrome.

Besides knowing your waist size, the screening itself is really quite simple. It can be done in any doctor's office and is given at many health fairs. You need to have your blood pressure taken (which I am in favor of writing down for future reference; I ask my patients to keep a little card in their wallet in order to track their blood pressure over time). Then you need a blood test for fasting sugar and blood lipids. The lipids test is for cholesterol, HDL cholesterol, and triglycerides. That's all there is to it. (It is not necessary to test for insulin levels, but if you are at risk, it is worth asking your doctor to do it.)

Fatal Flaws

The most obvious cause of cardio-metabolic syndrome is weight gain, based on the circumference of the abdomen. Eating as little as fifty to one hundred excess calories a day can accumulate into a significant weight gain and contribute greatly to your risk of this disease.

A particular type of diet can also make you susceptible to cardio-metabolic syndrome: one that is high in processed sugars. A diet high in processed sugar can cause elevations of blood pressure, blood sugar, and triglycerides, and reductions in HDL cholesterol. In other words, it can lead to all aspects of this syndrome.

Obviously, inactivity is another contributing cause of cardio-metabolic syndrome. Excessive intakes of calories and sugars that are not counterbalanced by exercise will result in weight gain and will aggravate the chemical abnormalities listed above.

However, there is one other major contributing factor of this syndrome: heredity. If your parents or close relatives have the conditions above, you are at higher genetic risk to develop cardio-metabolic syndrome, too. So if one of your parents had diabetes, hypertension (elevated blood pressure), high triglycerides or low HDL cholesterol levels, then there is a fairly good chance that you have a hereditary risk of cardio-metabolic syndrome. If your family is susceptible, you should take extra care with your lifestyle.

Now, I know some people are reading this and thinking, "So what? I have a few extra pounds around the waist. What's the big deal? Who doesn't? My blood pressure is borderline elevated but it doesn't hurt me—I mean I have no pain. Oh, so my triglycerides are a little high. What are they anyway? But my HDL cholesterol is low. Low cholesterol is good, right?"

These are all arguments I get from patients who would prefer simply not knowing. They want to justify continuing to eat junk food on the couch while they vegetate in front of the TV.

But here's why knowing about this condition is important: cardio-metabolic syndrome is lethal. Once these conditions start to occur, you are already well on your way to a coffin. In fact, your risk of dying from a cardiovascular condition is increased by 75 percent! That doesn't sound very harmless to me.

It would be easy for me, and every doctor, if all illnesses had obvious symptoms, such as the ones that really catch patients' attention: bleeding and pain. If every time you had a candy bar you started to bleed from your colon, it might get your attention. If every time you sat on the couch for an hour you developed chest pain, it would not be difficult to initiate life changes.

Unfortunately, cardio-metabolic syndrome has no symptoms in its earlier phases. It sneaks up on you just like the weight around your waist. The first symptom that you notice could very well be a lethal heart attack. By the time most people are aware of this syndrome, it is relatively advanced. Aggressive lifestyle changes are needed before it becomes too late.

Compare this condition to cigarette smoking (which is an unhealthy habit that I am in no way recommending). Cigarettes increase your risk of dying by 60 percent, so cardio-metabolic syndrome is a more serious risk factor than smoking! There are campaigns to remove smoking from all public places, yet no one has started an anti-cardio-metabolic syndrome campaign. No one has said, "Let's remove candy machines from all public places." Well, consider this the start of that campaign.

Almost without a doubt, you or someone close to you is suffering from cardio-metabolic syndrome. It is a deadly, ticking time bomb of a condition. However, it can be reversed. I did it, as did many of my patients. But before you change your condition, you have to change your mind and realize that sustained, healthy lifestyle habits are the cure.

Your mind is what provides you with an identity. You may see yourself as an inactive person who has some extra poundage in the middle, but you need to change that perception of yourself in small steps. You need to change from the person who gobbles any garbage food like a starving dog to a person who cares for your body and health and believes in the differences you are making.

Follow the Globe's Best Diet and you will perceive of yourself as a health-conscious person who selects natural, delicious food. You will become that active person that your mind wants you to be. Start to formulate a new, better perception of your body and your health. It will start as a thought but, with practice, will become a natural, effortless habit. Then, before you know it, you will have changed—and perhaps saved—your life.

Chapter 6: Affecting Change

Most readers probably picked up this book looking for an easy answer to weight loss that does not require any change or effort on their part. They really had no intention of changing anything at first.

Chapters two, three, and four should have planted a seed in your mind that change is essential. You and the rest of America are headed down a path of obesity, malnutrition, disease, and poisonous eating. The health consequences are expanding at a faster rate as obesity continues to spread. Change is necessary now; it is the only way to combat the epidemic. Your mind must prepare you for change. Mentally, you must find the motivation and the energy to initiate the action phase. This is when the concept builds momentum and the first behavioral changes occur.

Over the next few chapters, I will reveal some of the diet options that will lead you to the goal of good health. I recommend that you read and savor every step. After you finish each chapter, start to implement the recommended changes immediately. They are what will guide you toward a better, leaner lifestyle.

Changing Your Mind—and Your Body
Of course, these changes are not only physical but psychological. There are certain character traits that you will need to practice and develop along the way: discipline, patience, and persistence, which all lead to higher self-worth.

To succeed in anything long-term, you need to develop

discipline, which was derived from Latin, meaning "to learn or instruct." The purpose of this book is to instruct you about healthy lifestyles and diet, and for you to learn to follow a certain code of conduct, self-control, and beneficial behavior. Once you adopt these steps and a certain pattern of action, they become habit, or ingrained behavior that occurs automatically. Won't that be nice? When you develop these habits by repeating the same healthy behaviors over and over again, they become easier and more acceptable to you; they become your way of life. Eventually, the positive effects you see and feel as a result will reinforce this behavior and motivate you to continue it.

One method to aid in habit development is affirmations, or statements of desirable intentions. Examples would be, "I will live a healthier life," "I will follow a better diet," or "I will exercise today." If you make these promises to yourself, they will serve as motivators in helping you to develop better lifestyle habits.

"Patience" also has its roots in Latin, meaning "to suffer." It would be wonderful if our goals were instantaneously met through small amounts of change. Unfortunately, to affect change requires effort and time. If you don't see immediate results, you may consider this process a form of "suffering." But I view a healthy, carbohydrate-restricted diet combined with an invigorating exercise program as an opportunity for a better life and more energy. The amazing foods you will eat that nature has to offer far surpass what the machines grind out. The energy that comes from not being weighed down by extra pounds or poisoned by bad foods will recharge you, and your newfound endurance will expand your life. Remember that it took many years of bad lifestyle choices for your body to become ill. The road to recovery will also take some time. Consider it a healthy, delicious journey that only gets better with each step.

Persistence is defined as "insisting repetitively." You must develop new habits, and these must be repeated daily until they become your way of living. You must consistently say no to unhealthy and lethal foods that are toxins to your body. As you gain an appreciation for the finer foods, the old habits will become extinguished and you will become healthier. That is the reward for persistence.

I have developed a habit of just saying no to bad foods. On a daily basis, people will offer me unhealthy snacks, usually junk rich in carbohydrates (I'm sure this happens to you, too, especially in the workplace). I persistently decline. If they ask why, I say I'm on a low-carbohydrate diet, which not only satisfies them but eventually gives them the idea to stop offering, accept "no" very quickly, or surprise me by bringing in some fresh fruit one day. By being persistent in your healthy habits, you may find that you are not only changing yourself but helping the people around you change, too.

Breaking down Barriers

Behavior patterns can be barriers to change. For some, emotional issues can prevent consistent improvement as they eat to provide comfort to themselves from emotional upset. Diet changes may work well during stable periods, but times of stress can thwart discipline. The treatment is to learn to cope with emotional turmoil in other ways, which can involve counseling, exercise, or a twelve-step program such as Overeaters Anonymous.

Other people eat out of boredom, and time spent at home is riddled with refrigerator trips. You must learn to avoid your eating environments. Walks around the block should replace walks to the refrigerator.

Others simply lack control. This can be constant or a case of a binge-eating disorder with periodic loss of control. For these people, the issue is more complicated. Control must start first in the supermarket: you cannot eat what you don't buy. Go with a list and avoid impulse buys. A change of environment may also be required. Get out of the house and exercise or get involved in healthy, fun activities. Avoid hunger with small, nutritious snacks so that feeling hungry doesn't lead to rapid binging and loss of control. Medications like Prozac are helpful for those with actual binge-eating disorders.

Dietary changes can be recommended by physicians; patients, now thinking they know what to do, simply comply with someone else's prescription (which usually lasts for a whole day or two after the doctor appointment). But the goal of this book is not compliance. The goal is adherence.

Adherence is sticking to a program because you know that it is the right thing for you. It is not like compliance, when you do something on someone else's orders. The Globe's Best Diet is for you because you believe and care about your health and your body, and you want to do what is best for yourself.

Affecting change provides you with an opportunity. Without change, you will remain stuck with the same unhealthy lifestyle. With change, you reopen the door to a world of delicious, natural foods and increased energy. Take advantage of that opportunity. Enjoy the change! Enjoy life!

Chapter 7: Irreplaceable Exercise

One of the most important aspects of any diet is exercise. In fact, it is probably the most essential component to long-term change and success.

I know that many of you looking for an easy way to lose weight may be tempted to skip this chapter and move on to the "quick fix." Without reading what's in here, however, any attempts that you make at weight loss will fail.

A lack of exercise is the number one lifestyle defect. There are more people who fail to exercise than there are those who smoke, drink alcohol excessively, or eat gluttonously. In fact, about 50 percent of all people are largely inactive. They do not even meet the minimum guidelines for necessary physical activity.

The consequence of all this inactivity is death. Physical inertia leads to at least two hundred fifty thousand deaths annually in the United States. Are you going to be one of them?

Getting Physical

Regular exercise has a plethora of benefits, all of which can save your life. It decreases the incidence of cardiovascular diseases, like heart attacks, strokes, and hypertension, and reduces the risk of diabetes and even some cancers (recent evidence shows a clear reduction in breast cancer among those who exercise).

Physical activity also improves mental health. It is a great stress reducer, mood enhancer, and also increases energy levels and endurance. It prevents osteoporosis and helps older patients maintain their mobility while decreasing their chance of disabilities and falls.

When it comes to exercise, more is better. The more you work out, the more benefits you will see. But why is exercise so important for weight? It really comes down to basic physics.

Think of it like the scale of justice: on one side is energy expenditure, on the other side, energy input. The difference between the two determines whether your weight will go up or down. You can fool yourself and the scale temporarily, but the long-term result will be the same.

A person's weight is determined by the net difference between calorie intake and calorie expenditure: calories in minus calories out equals weight change. Ideally, you want the calories you get rid of to be more than those you take in. You can achieve this in several ways. One is by greatly decreasing the calories you eat. This gets tricky, though, because fasting triggers hunger and the weight loss process actually becomes painful.

Alternatively, you can greatly increase the calories out through vigorous exercise. However, if you are heavily overeating, you may have to do enormous amounts of exercise to counterbalance the calories you consume, so this can be a very frustrating solution. I see many people who spend hours at the gym, only to gorge on food later. They make no progress in spite of their massive efforts.

Most people underestimate their calorie intake and overestimate the effects of their exercise. It can become quite annoying and time-consuming, not to mention painful, to spend an hour on a treadmill to work off half a dozen cookies that you shouldn't have eaten in the first place.

So the best solution is a combination. You want to decrease your caloric intake by about five hundred calories a day, and supplement that with around three hundred *negative* calories burned off by moderate exercise. This will result in a net loss of eight hundred calories daily and an average weight loss of two to three pounds per week. If a pill was proven to do that, I bet many of you would buy it!

Slow and Steady

That brings us to the topic of the speed of weight loss. You see many products guaranteeing rapid weight loss: "Lose twenty-one pounds in twenty-one days." This type of claim is pure malarkey—and if you fall for it, you are fooling only yourself. If you lose twenty-one pounds in twenty-one days, it will all be fluid weight, not fat. You may even lose muscle mass. The scale has deceived you, and the process has harmed your body. Instead of losing unhealthy fat, you lost essential fluids and muscle.

Don't try to beat the system. It is much easier to lose fluid, and people will naturally take the easy route. Some may try going to a sauna, where the body can lose five to ten pounds of fluid under these extreme conditions. But as soon as they drink liquids to replenish, the weight will return. Some people try to take diuretics to expel liquids, use cathartics to induce bowel movements, or follow fad diets that deplete their body of fluids. The end result is the same: no true weight loss, just a temporary high when the scale shows a smaller number for a few hours or days.

But that euphoric feeling will be removed when the fluids are returned to your body and the weight is rapidly regained. Rapid weight loss like that is always followed by rapid weight gain. These measures will not produce any long-term benefits to your system—not a bit. But there is a great amount of potential harm.

Very rapid weight loss can destroy essential muscle and other vital structures. The subject has been studied quite carefully and in depth, and the conclusion is: if you want to lose fat and not fluid or muscle, then a certain amount of nutrition is necessary to maintain proper bodily function. Protein is the most essential of these components, so a low-fat, high-carb diet will not supply what you need. With a proper level of protein, caloric, and nutrient intake, it is possible to lose weight—but at a rate of no faster than two to three pounds of fat per week! If you are losing more that that, it is all fluid and essential muscle.

There are some rare exceptions. In the first week or two of a new diet, some people may lose five to seven pounds. They may have had a lot of fat and carbohydrate stores to lose, but some of it may also be fluids and water weight. There are occasionally people able to restrict calories and maintain very vigorous exercise programs who may lose weight more rapidly, but as the body gets severely deficient in calories, they might start to break down muscle in addition to fat in order to achieve a caloric balance.

On a long-term basis, a two- to three-pound weekly weight loss is the only reasonable and achievable goal. Anything more is dangerous and ineffective in the long run. But if you think about it, these numbers really begin to add up. Let's say you maintain an exercise program of walking two miles a day, therefore burning off 340 calories. If you also restrict your intake by 200 calories a day through eliminating some processed carbohydrates like cookies, candies, etc., your body will have a negative balance of 500 calories. These modest changes will remove one pound of fat weekly—or fifty-two pounds in a year!

The Dreaded Scale

Too much focus on the scale every day can cause you to do exactly the wrong thing. Many people will start to restrict their fluids, like water, so that the reading appears better that day, which, in turn, makes them feel better emotionally. In the long run, however, water depletion promotes fat gain, which will make you feel worse physically. In fact, if you drink lots of water, it may temporarily provide or accentuate the fullness that is achieved from proper diet, and you may eat less.

On the other hand, there are people who make the mistake of never getting on the scale at all. This is a very bad habit. I see many patients who haven't weighed themselves in months or years, and are shocked at the result. If you weigh yourself regularly, you can fine-tune your intake and make adjustments more rapidly when your caloric balance is out of whack. Think about it: it may not be nice to see, but it is much easier to treat a three-pound weight gain than that of twenty-five pounds.

In studies of those who have successfully lost weight, about half had weighed themselves daily. Those who stopped weighing themselves usually regained the weight. My advice? Lose weight with your eyes open, not shut.

Calories Count

If you are able to truly change the balance of energy, and not just the balance of fluids, you will achieve real weight loss. Forget about adjusting your scale! Even minor adjustments of caloric intake over time can have profound effects. But if the balance is off even slightly, then it will add up.

If your take in twenty calories more per day than you put out, over one year's time you will gain two pounds. So while cutting twenty calories a day may seem like a minute change, the long-term consequences can be huge. Of course, it requires patience to see the results of small changes.

Over a decade, an extra twenty calories daily will result in a thirty- to forty-pound weight gain. That's all it takes. One extra cookie a day can put you in the danger zone.

But look at the reverse. If you take in twenty fewer calories instead of overeating by twenty calories a day, over time the results will be fabulous. Small but sustainable changes will trump dramatic, unsustainable changes every time.

How long can you eat just cabbage soup anyway? Maybe you can stomach it a month or two. But how long can you continue your habit of taking a walk around the block? How long can you go without the weekly purchase of junk food at the supermarket or that extra cookie before bed? These are livable changes that have a chance of becoming long-term habits, lifestyles, and parts of your identity. You can determine who you want to be: an unenergetic blob or an active, vibrant person? You make the choice—then make the changes.

Walking to Win ...

It's time to go with the winners. There was a study called the National Weight Registry, which evaluated people who had successfully lost and kept off more than 10 percent of their body weight. These people had lost an average of around sixty-five pounds and kept it off for an average of five-and-a-half years. How did these winners keep off the weight? Was it the cabbage soup diet? Not likely! An increase in physical activity was reported by 81 percent of them.

You may think that the increase in exercise was fairly dramatic to achieve such results, but let's break it down. Women expended around 2,500 kcal a week and men burned off even more, a total of 3,300 kcal a week. What does that mean in terms of activity? If you walk a mile, you burn off 170 kcal. So, in distance, the women were walking close to fifteen miles a week or about two miles a day. Most people walk a mile in around fifteen to twenty minutes, so that involved thirty to forty minutes of walking a day. The men were walking twenty miles a week, which is closer to three miles a day. That's an investment of forty-five minutes to an hour of exercise each day. That doesn't sound so bad, right? It's a very reasonable goal—and well worth it when you consider the results.

It should be no surprise, then, that walking is my most recommended weight loss tool. How much should you walk? Well, how much do you want to lose? If you need to lose a lot of weight, then the more you walk, the better. You don't have to jog; just take a little more time to walk it off.

When I am in serious weight-loss mode, I walk eight miles a day, or around forty to fifty miles a week. I walk a mile in fifteen minutes and go for a one-hour walk twice a day. Occasionally, I walk one hour in one direction then turn around and go back, doubling my efforts.

For those physically handicapped by weight, just ten minutes of walking can be a strain. That's okay. Even ten minutes is enough to count as activity. If that's all that you can do to start out with, then do those ten minutes. If you can do it more than once a day, even better. You can add up your exercise time to achieve the general thirty-minute goal.

Some people use a pedometer during their walks to help them measure the number of steps they have taken daily. If you'd like to be that precise, I recommend that you start with five thousand steps a day. If you can build up to ten thousand, then you will really accelerate your weight loss.

...And Playing to Win

Of course, there are many alternatives to walking for physical activity. For those who are very inactive and may want companionship when they exercise, walking a dog is acceptable. Dog walking is slower-paced since these pets don't understand the concept of exercise; they are more interested in sniffercise. Nonetheless, even this activity is better than none.

Many other everyday actions qualify as moderate exercise. Some may be hobbies that you actually enjoy, such as carpentry, gardening, and working on your car. Also, many household chores involve physical activity, like mowing the lawn, washing the car, mopping, vacuuming, and sweeping. There are even some activities that provide more exercise than you'd think. I was surprised to find that many studies ranked bowling, fishing (if standing), ping pong, sailing, and tai chi as forms of moderate exercise. Even fun activities like tossing around a Frisbee or playing with your children can count as moderate physical activity. There are so many choices, in fact, that excuses for a lack of exercise are futile, yet everybody seems to come up with a few.

You don't have to belong to a gym to get variety in your exercise. You can make it fun by mixing it up. If you walk, vary the pace, sometimes jogging, sometimes running. Or choose a route with a different view. You can also swim, bike, rollerblade, or dance to spice things up.

If you do belong to a gym, you can walk or jog on a treadmill or on a track. You can use a stair-climber, exercise bike, or elliptical machine. You can add rowing equipment or, for a really killer workout, use the cross-country ski machines. You can do all of the above.

Since I live in Florida, one of my favorite forms of exercise is a walk on the beach. (A park will do just as well if it's in your neighborhood.) I also like jogging on a treadmill in front of a television screen (or three) at the gym since the multitasking prevents boredom.

For people who already suffer from arthritis, or for anyone in general who has access to a pool, swimming or exercising in water are great, less strenuous ways to be active. These options reduce calories quickly, and because the water provides resistance, simple movements can count as exercise. The water's buoyant effect absorbs the shock to achy joints. There is one caveat that comes along with water exercise: for some reason, it is slightly less effective at burning off fat than other forms of physical activity. It could be that since one of fat's functions is to protect the body from heat loss, and submersion in water can cause that; the body may try to compensate by retaining fat. Still, using a pool is best for arthritis sufferers, and some people just enjoy it more, which is a very important consideration.

Get Off the Sofa and Start Exercising!

If you don't enjoy your exercise, it will be murder to keep up. But one of the key factors to continuing physical activity is simply to start it! I can think of a hundred reasons on any given day why I can't exercise, and through the years I have heard them all repeated to me by the patients in my office.

A usual one is, "Doc, I just don't have the time." But this is a really wimpy excuse. You have time for whatever you make a priority in your life. If you really wanted to do it, you would find the time or make the time. I have patients who get up at 4:00 a.m. to exercise and those who go for a walk on their lunch hour. Personally, I work a twelve-hour day and still manage to find time for daily exercise. It is amazing to me how many people don't have time to exercise, but do have an extra three hours to spare sitting in front of the TV or surfing the Internet in the evening. Put a treadmill in front of your television set, if that's what it takes! Another popular excuse is, "I don't have a pool or access to a gym." Neither of these things is required. Walking doesn't involve a gym, and even though I am not a huge fan of home exercise equipment because it often becomes a dust collector for many people, it can provide convenient, intermittent outlets for exercise. Many pieces of home gym equipment for sale by their owners are listed as "used" but are in brand-new condition! This tells you something about how often they are utilized. Buy one at a good price and remember that even short bursts of exercise can improve long-term weight loss.

I've shared with you some of my patients' favorite sayings. Now let me tell you a saying that we have in the medical profession: if you can't find time for exercise, then you had better find time for disease. And, don't worry, that disease will come find you.

The Health Effects of Exercise

Beyond weight loss, there are additional benefits to regular exercise. It has a definite effect on lowering blood pressure—reducing it an average of three-and-a-half points. Blood pressure also drops proportionately to ongoing weight loss, as we have already seen.

Weight-bearing exercise, like walking and jogging, strengthens the bones. Those who regularly exercise in these ways are less likely to get osteoporosis, which, in itself, can become a vicious cycle. Once you develop osteoporosis and have profound spinal curvature, it can be very difficult to do much weight-bearing exercise.

Regular activity also greatly reduces the risk of diabetes. Both fat and sugar are burned off and your body retains its ability to handle sugar loads (though it does not develop resistance to the effects of insulin). If you already have diabetes, exercise will lower your average blood sugar reading (hemoglobin A1C) by 0.5–1.0 percent—and a lower reading will help to prevent complications associated with the disease.

Studies have also shown that exercise helps to reduce the chances of developing cancer of the breast and colon, although exactly how is not yet understood.

In addition, physical exercise can have excellent psychological effects. It releases endorphins, part of the natural morphine system, that cause a calming, relaxed sensation, help to lower stress levels, and elevate your mood. Depression is a condition that can definitely be improved by exercise, and I have personally found it invaluable for handling high-stress situations.

In a comparison of lean exercisers to lean sedentary people, those who are sedentary are still at a 50 percent higher risk of dying, even though they appear "fit." The risk is even greater for obese people. If you are obese but don't keep up an active lifestyle, your risk of dying is two-and-a-half times greater. So the point is that, regardless of what you weigh, you are far better off exercising, even if weight loss is not your target or you don't lose significant weight doing it. You will still achieve significant health benefits and live longer.

How Much is Enough?

How much activity do you need to maintain in order to achieve the benefits of exercise and define yourself as active? About three-and-a-half hours a week (or about thirty minutes a day) is enough to give you life-prolonging effects. If you exercise less than that, there are still life-extending benefits, but a slightly less amount. So any bit helps.

I recommend setting your sights on exercising seven days a week for thirty minutes daily. Every now and then you will have a legitimate reason not to exercise on a given day. If you net five days out of a week, you are doing reasonably well. This means you don't miss more than two consecutive days—because by the time you get to your third day without exercise, your metabolic rate already starts to slow. Your body starts to release more insulin and the weight-gain process resumes. That's why it's important to keep those activity vacations to two days or less.

If you change your exercise from something brisk, like walking (moderate activity), to a more vigorous activity, like jogging, then even more life-extending benefits can be achieved. In fact, it actually requires less exercise time if you choose vigorous exercise: only twenty minutes three times weekly to achieve a risk about 5 percent lower than the moderate exerciser. (That will lower your risk by 55 percent compared to an inactive person.)

If you are really an exercise nut like me and do both moderate and vigorous exercise, then you achieve the lowest risk of all, dropping it by another third. You lower your risk of death to only 30 percent compared to those who are inactive.

How can you possibly do all that? As an example, I go for a walk on the beach or in the park most days, but three days a week I crank it up in the gym and push myself on a treadmill. The different sceneries help me avoid the boredom that can come from being in the gym all the time, and when I exercise on the treadmill, I have a TV in front of me so I can catch up on the latest news, sports, or if you like, soap operas. (If you are really serious about weight loss, you should substitute active endeavors for your TV time. People who are successful at losing weight and keeping it off average less than ten hours a week in front of the boob tube.)

The argument for exercise is particularly persuasive when you look at it like this: burning about one thousand calories a week through exercise will decrease your chances of dying by 20 to 40 percent. In terms of walking, that's about seven miles a week— which is not a long way to go to increase your life.

A sample workout program is listed below in Table 2. This program should be individually modified based upon your exercising preferences. If, for example, you prefer biking or playing racquetball, then you may substitute an equal exercise time for your preferred activity.

Table 2 Sample Workout Program

	Fitness	Maximum Weight Loss	Peak Fitness
Sunday	30 minute walk	1 hour walk	
Monday	30 minute walk	1 hour walk	
Tuesday	30 minute walk	1 hour walk	
Wednesday			20 minute jog
Thursday	30 minute walk	1 hour walk	
Friday	30 minute walk	1 hour walk	
Saturday			20 minute jog

Weighing in on Weight Training

Should you try weight training? The answer is yes and no on that one. To be honest, I have been lifting weights since 1984 and so I am in favor of it overall. I have also seen many people working out in the gym through the years, so I know what works—and I know that if you are trying to lose a lot of weight right now, weight lifting should not be your priority.

First of all, weight training is an inefficient way of burning calories. It involves brief exercise followed by minutes of rest. For weight loss, more continuous exercise, such as walking or biking, is preferable.

Secondly, lifting weights sends your body mixed messages. While you are telling it to burn off fat and sugar, you are simultaneously telling it to build more muscle. The result is a change in body composition without any net change in weight.

Thirdly, where are the studies? Although I have seen plenty of research linking aerobic activities, like walking or jogging, to weight loss, I have not seen any good studies documenting sustained weight loss through weight training.

Finally, there are my own observations and experiences. With all my years in the gym, I have yet to meet someone who maintained significant weight loss through weight training alone. Yet I see a majority of overweight people, especially men, on the wrong side of the gym lifting weights. I don't understand their obsession with the bench press. Why would these men want bigger breasts?

Of course, there is another side of the coin. After all, there must be some reason I have been weight training for the last twenty-four years, right? It is okay to make weight training a *part* of your exercise program. As I've mentioned, people on protein- and calorie-deprived diets lose fat and sugar, but also muscle mass at times. Muscle is your metabolic factory; if you continually lose it, you will slow your metabolic rate and weight loss will become increasingly difficult. (This process happens not only with dieting, but also with aging. It turns out that your muscle mass peaks around age twenty-five and you lose 10 percent of it every decade thereafter. So, by sixty-five, you will have lost 40 percent of your muscle mass and your metabolic rate will be 40 percent less. Many patients have realized that they eat far less than they did when they were younger, yet they gain weight. The reason for this is decreased metabolic rate—and diminished activity also plays a role.) To counteract this loss of muscle from both dieting and aging, you can use weight training. It can reverse the loss of muscle and help restore your metabolism.

However, weight training, like any exercise, can be dangerous and injury can occur, particularly with heavy weights. I recommend that you start with a weight at which you can comfortably do fifteen to twenty-five repetitions. If you want to develop strength in addition to tone, you can add a slightly heavier weight for the second set, one at which you can comfortably do ten to fifteen repetitions. For your final set, you can use an even heavier weight if strengthening is desired; shoot for a weight at which you can do five to eight repetitions. (anything below five repetitions dramatically increases the risk of injury).

To focus on weight loss through weight training as part of your routine, stick mostly to working out the large muscle groups: thighs, chest, biceps, triceps, and back. Back exercises must be done with extreme caution, especially squats. (I do not recommend squats; the injury risk is very high and a lower back injury could be devastating to your exercise regimen.) It is always best to learn the proper technique for each exercise you choose. Improper techniques increase your risk of injury, so get initial instruction from a qualified personal trainer.

A sample weight training program is listed below in Table 3. This program should be specifically modified to the individual based on any physical problems or limitations.

Table 3- Sample Weight Training Program

	Exercise	Sets	Reps
Chest	Bench Press	2-3	15,10, 5
Shoulders	Dumbbell Laterals	2	15,10
Back	Pull Downs	2	15,10
Biceps	Barbell Curls	2-3	15,10,5-8
Triceps	Triceps Push Down	2	15,10
Quadriceps	Leg Extension	2	15,10
Hamstring	Leg Curls	2	15,10
Calf	Calf Raises	2	15,10
Abdominals	Basic Crunch	2	15-25
	Elbow alt Knees	2	15-25
	Leg Lateral Raises	2	15-25

We all know that lifting weights makes your body look great, but there is a little known factor about weight training that I want to share with you. Most people want to maintain their independence in life, which becomes particularly important as they reach old age. Older people exercise to stay fit, often doing cardiovascular training that involves treadmills, stationary bikes, etc. However, what actually determines independence in old age is not cardiovascular fitness but being able to perform the tasks of daily living. An older person may strain a weak muscle just by reaching for a can of soup, and the most important muscles are those in the hip that are used to get someone out of a chair or bed. Once these muscles deteriorate to the point that someone can't perform these simple tasks, they can no longer live independently. For this reason, weight training that pinpoints certain muscle groups makes a lot of sense for senior citizens, regardless of their weight-loss goals.

It's All Starting to Sink In

There are some signs that people are finally getting the message: regular physical activity has had a slight upturn in the last five years. The percentage of women exercising regularly has increased from 43 to 47 percent. Men haven't increased quite as much; 48 percent exercised regularly in 2001 and it went up to a total of 50 percent in 2006. Those in the higher risk groups for obesity, such as black women, are also catching on, increasing regular exercise from 31 to 36 percent. Unfortunately, this still puts them far behind many other categories—and, statistically, they are the most obese demographic group.

You don't have to be fat. You don't have to be an unenergetic blob. You don't have to feel emotionally poor. You don't have to develop the illnesses brought on by weight gain. You *can* change. But you have to change your mind first.

Step one is that you have to *want* to change. Then your mind must change its perception of yourself. You need to think of yourself as a physically active person and start with small steps to demonstrate that behavior. Make a plan to start some type of daily physical activity, no matter how small. Gradually build on that activity until you believe in yourself and incorporate it as part of your lifestyle.

Activity does not have to be painful or unpleasant; it can help you enjoy some of the basic pleasures in life. A simple walk in the park or on the beach can produce great physical and mental benefits. For those who have enjoyed biking, racquetball, or swimming in the past, by all means return to what you love. This will make activity effortless and enjoyable.

Leave yourself reminders on the refrigerator and elsewhere to participate in your activity of choice. Write a sticky note on your

TV set or computer and also keep a log there to document your daily exercise times or the steps you've made.

Whatever activity you choose, DO choose activity. It is an essential part of your program for health. Start today. Make it a habit. Then make it your lifestyle.

Chapter 8: Relearning How—and What—to Eat

We all learn how to put food in our mouths when we're babies. That's a simple case of starvation or survival. But now it's time to really learn *how* to eat properly—and I'm not talking about table manners!

Meal Size and Frequency

The Japanese have a solution to weight gain, and Okinawa, an island in Japan, is famous for longevity. Here is one of their secrets: they practice the principle of *hara hachi bu,* which means, "Eat until you are eight out of ten parts full." If you can incorporate this concept into your lifestyle, it will have long-lasting effects. That does not mean to go hungry. It means always leave a little room. Do not eat until you are bloated and uncomfortable. That just makes sense, right?

There are other ways to adjust your diet to provide lean nutrition without having to experience hunger. One such essential concept for weight loss is meal frequency. Most obese people are in the habit of skipping meals. They believe that eating less frequently is the solution to losing weight. However, studies have shown that exactly the opposite is true.

The original studies were carried out on rats and showed that if you fed them once daily, they would gobble up all of the food immediately and gain weight. If you took the same amount of food and spread it out over different times of day, the rats would eat less and lose weight.

While the rats seem to have this eating pattern down pat,

most *people* still have trouble understanding this concept—but the same has been shown to be true for us.

The difference is in metabolism. If the body waits a prolonged period of time for food, it interprets this as a starvation condition, which immediately slows metabolism. When new food is introduced, the body tries to store it as fat as quickly as possible to prepare for future starvation modes.

When the body has frequent food sources, however, it burns them almost as soon as they are consumed. There is no slowing of the metabolism. In fact, each time new food is eaten, there is a one- to two-hour increase in metabolic rate. This surge in metabolism is repeated many times daily in one who nibbles.

Want a surefire way to get fat? Obese people typically starve themselves all day and eat dinner very late, when they are ravenously hungry. They eat quickly and without control, which worsens the problem. The brain registers food intake thirty to sixty minutes after eating, but during that delay period, an uncontrollably hungry person continues to eat. That person therefore overeats beyond being full and becomes bloated. Then the body attempts to store as much of that food as possible.

Many obese people will go to bed shortly thereafter, and that inactivity promotes more weight gain. They awaken still bloated and skip breakfast, continuing what the body perceives as starvation conditions until, like the rats, they binge again before bed. If this describes your lifestyle, you are doomed to failure on any diet unless you change your eating pattern.

Most successful weight-loss programs involve frequent meals. Breakfast, no matter how small, is essential. Typically, a diet that involves frequent, smaller snacks is recommended. This usually involves eating about five to six times daily so that each snack stimulates the metabolism and promotes energy burning. Weight Watchers, which is a reasonable program, instructs people that they cannot lose weight if they don't eat enough. Your may find that ironic, but if you want to maintain control of your hunger, you must give your body a steady stream of healthy nutrition. Loss of control will only thwart your efforts.

The Globe's Best Diet that I am recommending involves frequent, healthy, and delicious snacks. No matter what the fads say, hunger is *not* a requirement for healthy eating.

Now we know how to eat. But what exactly should we be putting in our bodies?

Debunking the Low-Fat Lie

Everywhere you look, so-called "experts" are touting "low-fat." Doctors preach it, and the food and advertising industries have jumped on the bandwagon. Many popular diets, including those recommended by medical associations, are based on the low-fat premise. Even your friends will vouch for the effectiveness of low-fat foods.

The facts, though, are quite different from what "everyone" says. As we all know, what is commonly believed to be valid is not always based on scientific truth. After all, the earth is not flat, although you would have been called a heretic for saying so in the Middle Ages. Similarly, the low-fat myth has been propagated as truth, and the public has bought into it. Well, it's high time we explore the *real* facts—and relearn how and what to eat.

The low-fat myth goes something like this: A low-fat diet is the healthiest. It will promote weight loss, lower your cholesterol (which is only partially true, by lowering good cholesterol) and decrease your chance of coronary artery disease (this one is probably not true, as we will discuss later).

The low-fat diet is not a fad that will die out anytime soon, though it should. You will most likely run into low-fat vigilantes for many decades to come—so it is important that you know its false foundations and have confidence in your lifestyle following The Globe's Best Diet instead.

As I stated in chapter two, the conclusions of the seven-country study conducted more than half a century ago formed the basis of our low-fat myth. The Cretan diet was determined to be ideal, so logically you'd think that the medical establishment would have recommended a diet like the Cretans. But that was not the case. The Cretan diet is *not* a low-fat diet! In fact, it was one of the highest-fat diets in the study.

Here is the typical Cretan diet (for simplicity, I have converted the daily intake from grams to ounces): (Table 4 below)

Table 4: Cretan Diet 1960

Fruit: 16 oz.
Bread: 13.3 oz.
Milk: 8.2 oz.
Vegetables: 6.7 oz.
Potatoes: 6.6 oz.
Edible fats (olives): 3.3 oz.
Meat: 1.22 oz.
Cereal: 1 oz.
Eggs: 0.87 oz.
Sugar: 0.7 oz.
Fish: 0.6 oz.
Cheese: 0.45 oz.
All Else: 3.7 oz.
Pastries: 0 oz.

As you can see, the number one food eaten by Cretans is fruit! If anything, the dietary recommendation made to Americans should have been to eat more fruit.

Crete is an island garden. It is plentiful in fruits, vegetables, nuts, and dairy products, but there is not much grazing. Beef and other meats are not readily available and are expensive, so Cretans do not consume very much red meat, only about one ounce a day, and get by with what they can grow in their gardens. Olives, which are quite plentiful, are their top product, and olive oil is used exclusively in all cooking and in dressings. It is olive oil, nuts, dairy products, and to a lesser extent, fish that are their main sources of fat. In fact, approximately 40–45 percent of their diet is fat!

So, why were we told to reduce fat to less than 30 percent? And just how did the low-fat diet come out of this study? If, after twenty-five years of scientific research into global lifestyles, they determined that a high-fat diet works best, why was its *exact opposite* recommended to the American public?

The answer is simple but unsavory: politics! In the 1950s, America had its population sold on a steak-and-potatoes mentality. Many Midwestern states were dependent on cattle farms for their livelihoods, so for medical authorities and scientists to recommend not eating beef would have been un-American. Therefore, the results of the study were softened: "Don't eat fat."

Isn't that different than "Don't eat beef"? Yes, it is extremely different! If you restrict your fat intake, you will cut down on things like nuts, olive oil, dairy products, and fish, which are all essential parts of the Cretan diet, the healthiest in the world.

Furthermore, the nonspecific recommendation was to avoid fat, and people had to eat something. Since fat and protein are often linked together in foods like meat, fish, and dairy, if you restrict fat, you also restrict protein. So if you can't eat fat or protein, carbohydrates are all that's left! And another word for carbohydrates is "sugar."

Americans have followed these recommendations; they were trying to live healthily, so they have been eating more and more sugar! Lots of it! This is an example of bad science. A good study provided helpful recommendations; then the results were twisted, totally altering the conclusion. We have gone from "Don't eat too much beef" to "Don't eat fish, nuts, dairy, or olive oil and eat tons of sugar." And we have the expanding waistlines to prove that eating all of those carbohydrates promotes weight gain.

In the next chapter, we'll see how a high-carbohydrate diet makes you fat and a high-fat diet does exactly the opposite.

Chapter 9: Carbohydrates Simplified

Most people think of sugar as table sugar, which is far from the truth. Sugar comes in many forms and under many names. Sugar is an energy packet. Its sole purpose is to provide energy for life—and if the body doesn't get enough, it can make its own through chemistry. Other than that, sugar by itself provides no nutrient value. If you consume more than your body burns on a daily basis, that excess energy intake will be stored as fat.

There are other compounds that the body treats in a similar way to table sugar (sucrose) but they have different names, such as fructose (fruit sugar) and maltose (malt-derived sugar). However, the general medical term for *all* sugars is carbohydrates. If you want to know if there is any sugar in what you are eating, read the label. The amount of carbohydrates will tell you the total amount of all sugars.

So, the big question is, are sugars bad? It really depends on the company they keep. By themselves, they only provide energy and make fat. Many foods have sugars combined with other essential nutrients, and this combination can be the essence of healthy living. If you eliminate these foods, your body will suffer in the long run from a higher incidence of disease.

The bottom line is that sugars are the foods that can be the most frivolously dangerous for weight gain, yet they can also be partnered with vitally important nutrition. You must choose carefully!

Sorting Your Sugars

How can you differentiate between foods with nutritious sugars and the fattening ones? The simplest explanation I can give you is the packaging. If your sugar comes in a box, a package, or a wrapper, you probably shouldn't be eating it. It is probably an energy-charged food that has little or no nutritional value. If what you have chosen looks like it came directly off the tree or from the ground, you are probably eating something charged with lots of additional nutrients.

There are, of course, more complex ways of differentiating the good carbohydrate foods from the bad. Two such measures that will help you distinguish are the glycemic index and the glycemic load.

The glycemic index is determined in a laboratory and measures how much blood sugar is elevated two hours after a standard carbohydrate meal is consumed. Usually this is compared to the elevation of sugar that occurs after eating white bread, which is given a reading of 100—though this reading may vary tremendously from lab to lab. Some labs compare the reading to glucose (pure sugar) instead. If labs use different references, you can get readings that differ by 40 percent. Some international labs use slightly different foods (for example, rice varies from country to country) and the result is readings that can be very inconsistent. In my examples, I will refer to the 2002 international table with white bread as 100 (if you are using a glucose table, your numbers will be about 40 percent lower).

A high glycemic index occurs if a food acts mostly like pure sugar and is absorbed more quickly into the blood. The blood sugar will rise quite high in response to its entry into the system—and such high readings powerfully stimulate insulin release and weight gain (we'll see the connection in the following chapter). Therefore, you do not want a food with a high glycemic index. The lower the glycemic index, the better the food is for you.

It has been shown that high glycemic index foods increase your chance of diabetes by about 37 percent over six years. Particular foods that increase this risk are: potatoes (cooked or french fried), white rice, white bread, and carbonated beverages. High glycemic index foods may also increase your risk of breast cancer, especially if you don't exercise, and are associated with higher risks of colon cancer.

On the other hand, low glycemic index foods delay the return of hunger. As the sugar is slowly absorbed, insulin is not stimulated, and the sugar remains in the safe range for prolonged periods. Subsequent food intake is decreased because people feel fuller. Diets with low glycemic index foods result in better fat and weight loss than those full of high glycemic index foods. It isn't so much a matter of how much you eat but the quality of your food that is vitally important.

The next indicator is glycemic load, which measures the total effect of a carbohydrate meal on the system. It is not only determined by the quality of the food that you eat but also by the quantity. It takes the glycemic index and multiples it by an average serving size to determine its overall effect on the system. (As you can imagine, an average serving size is a variable amount. My average serving size may be different than yours, and an average American serving size might be quite supersized when compared to a Chinese portion.)

Keep in mind that these numbers are rough guides, especially in some instances. For example, carrots have been maligned as a high glycemic index vegetable and carbohydrate-restricted diets, such as Atkins, have recommended avoiding them, even though they are healthy. But it turns out that the old measures of glycemic index on carrots were probably inaccurate, with an average of 70 and a reading as high as 132. The most recent report on carrots shows a glycemic index of only 32.

How many carrots do you normally eat? For me, one would be a lot—and because of that small quantity, the glycemic load is 1. In other words, the total glycemic load is small because of a small portion size. On the other hand, if you eat a four-ounce bagel, you will have both a high glycemic index (103) and a high glycemic load (50). That is equal to the load of fifty carrots. Obviously, the bagel will cause surging insulin and more profound effects on your system. So, of the two measures, the glycemic load is more important.

Another example is an apple, which has a glycemic index of 40 and a glycemic load of 4.

Compare that to a six-ounce serving of pasta with a glycemic index of 81 and a glycemic load of 27. After eating the pasta, you will be hungry again in two hours; keep repeating that diet, and you will be fat in no time. Remember, too, that this is based on an average portion size. When I was in danger of almost developing cardio-metabolic syndrome, a six-ounce portion of pasta would have been an appetizer for me. Most Italian restaurants in the United States serve about double that size as an entree. Now, when I do eat pasta, my portion is about three ounces and I eat it with a large salad, lots of vegetables, and a meat or clam sauce.

Foods in their natural state have lower glycemic index numbers. Mother Nature packages natural sugars with healthy fiber and surrounds them with vitamins, nutrients, and natural antioxidants. These foods are more slowly absorbed because the fiber acts as a slow release mechanism for the sugars, which means that the amount of insulin released is minimized. Therefore, weight gain is also minimized, as is that secondary hunger that comes after a sugar rush. You feel fuller and free from hunger longer.

On the other hand, processed foods remove Mother Nature's packaging. The fiber components are stripped away, along with those essential vitamins, nutrients, and antioxidants. These foods are often white in color, such as white bread, rice, potatoes, and pasta. Instead of being enclosed in Mother Nature's colorful packaging, they are wrapped in plastic or come in cardboard. Sure, their concentrated sugars may taste great, but they are empty calories that have no nutritional value other than the sugar that is rushed into your bloodstream, causing an intense insulin surge. Fat is immediately stored and, two to three hours later, your sugar drops lower and you find yourself back at the candy machine looking for another rush.

Here are selected examples of glycemic index and glycemic load using the 2002 international tables. Source International Table of Glycemic Index and Glycemic Load Values: 2002." *American Journal of Clinical Nutrition* 76, no. 1 (July 2002): 5–56

Table 5: Glycemic Index and Load (based on a white bread reference):

Food Glycemic Index/Portion Size (ounces)/Glycemic Load

Food	Glycemic Index	Portion Size(Oz)	Glycemic Load
Pastries/cakes			
Chocolate Cake	54	4	20
Croissant	96	2	17
Doughnut	76	1.5	17
Blueberry Muffin	84	2	17
Pancake	96	2.5	39
Waffle	109	2	20
Pop-Tarts	109	1.5	25
Breads			
Bagel	103	2	25
Rye bread	58	2	10
Wheat bread	74	2	20
White bread	100	2	20
Seven-grain bread	79	2	16
Cereals			
All-Bran cereal	53	2	18
Cheerios	106	2	30
Corn Flakes	130	2	48
Coco Pops	110	2	40
Cream of Wheat	105	2	44
Rice Krispies	117	2	44
Special K	98	2	28

Food	Glycemic Index	Portion Size(Oz)	Glycemic Load
Muesli	94	2	34
Oat Bran(raw)	72	2	12
Porridge	83	8	17
Honey(for flavor)	78	1	12

Dairy
Ice Cream(low-fat)	67	2	6
Whole milk	38	8	3
Skim milk	46	8	3
Plain Yogurt	51	8	3
Yogurt with fruit	44	2	18
Soy milk	63	9	8

Beverages
Coca-Cola	76	8	14
Smoothie	48	8	14
Apple juice	55	8	12
Tomato juice	54	8	4
Orange juice	81	8	12
Gatorade	111	8	12

Fruit
Apple	52	4	6
Banana	74	4	11
Cherries	66	4	8
Plum	34	4	3
Raisins	91	2	28

Vegetables
Green peas	55	3	4
Sweet corn	78	3	8

Food	Glycemic Index	Portion Size(Oz)	Glycemic Load
Baked potato	121	5	17
French fries	107	5	22
Sweet potato	87	5	17
Beans			
Baked beans	69	5	7
Kidney beans	39	5	7
Lentils	42	5	5
Entrees			
Pizza(supreme)	43	3	7
White spaghetti	64	6	21
Wheat spaghetti	53	6	19
Macaroni	64	6	22
White rice	91	5	23
Brown rice	79	5	18
Green pea soup	94	8	27
Snacks			
Mars bar	89	2	25
Snickers bar	59	2	15
Cashews	32	2	4
Popcorn	103	2	24
Pretzel	119	2	32
Cracker	90	2	22
Cookie	85	2	17

I'd like to add a few observations about the information above. Breakfast is the most dangerous meal for high glycemic index and load since some of the highest foods are bagels, croissants, waffles, pancakes, doughnuts, and processed cereals. On the other hand, skipping breakfast altogether is a bad idea. In a recent study of people who were successful at losing and maintaining large amounts of weight, 78 percent ate breakfast regularly. The trick is to make reasonable breakfast choices.

Interestingly, dairy products have fairly low glycemic indexes and loads. Low-fat yogurt or cottage cheese might be a good breakfast alternative, as are oat bran and porridge. The fiber in oat bran is more effective at lowering cholesterol than many wheat bran cereals; the effects are modest, however (about a 4 percent drop), and caution must be exercised as to not overdo carbohydrate intake. Most fruits are low in glycemic index and load (with the exception of raisins) and make an excellent breakfast.

Of the snack foods, popcorn and pretzels rate poorly. Nuts (my personal favorite) have a glycemic load of only 4.

Potatoes are among the worst, whether baked or fried. Pizza isn't as bad as many people might expect (especially because adding a lot of toppings to white bread will slow the sugar absorption).

As for beverages, cola and Gatorade are worse than natural juices. It is has been shown that colas increase your blood pressure in addition to your weight, and diet colas are associated with elevated blood pressure (exactly how is unclear, but diet sodas are sweetened with artificial chemicals that have undetermined effects on the body's metabolic system). You are far better off with natural beverages like water, juice, green and black tea, or even coffee (tea and coffee have not been shown to elevate blood pressure).

In addition to their low glycemic index, whole grain products may also have additional protective effects: higher intake has been associated with lowering the risk of stroke by half. Other cardiovascular diseases are also reduced by careful ingestion of whole grain products. If you are going to eat a carbohydrate, you might as well eat one that has some additional benefit!

Americans still don't get it, though. We eat, on average, fifty-three pounds of bread a year. America's favorite by far is white bread, the most popular types of which remove fibers and add processed sugars for taste.

Of all the foods, empty carbohydrates are the most expendable. If you desire a lean and healthy body, it is these foods that you must navigate through most carefully. If you choose your carbohydrates wisely, you will be rewarded not only with natural, flavorful foods, but also with boundless amounts of essential nutrients and a healthy body. If you waste your carbohydrate foods on empty sugar, you will face life with a fat and malnourished body that is ripe for the development of disease.

"High" Risk

There is a direct correlation between the amount of high glycemic index foods eaten and the development of diabetes. This is not just a theory; there are facts to support it: high glycemic foods cause diabetes!

A high glycemic load has other implications, too. For one, the higher your glycemic load, the lower your good (HDL) cholesterol. It is associated with an increased risk of cardiovascular disorders—in some people, that increase can be as much as 47 percent. That means a much higher risk of dying from heart attacks and strokes, all from taking in a high-sugar diet. We were told to cut down on fat (and therefore eat more carbohydrates) to prevent heart attacks, yet the reverse is true!

Low glycemic index foods have the opposite effect. People who consume whole grain products, like cereal, are actually protected from illness, reducing their chances of diabetes by 20 percent and decreasing their risk of stroke. One cup of whole grain cereal a day decreases heart failure by 28 percent (though other good sources of these fibers are dark breads, such as wheat, rye, or pumpernickel).

Thin people benefit even more, reducing their risk of developing cardiovascular disease in half by sticking to whole grain products. If thin people were to consume high glycemic load foods, they would double their risk of developing cardiovascular disease.

As you can see, the type of sugar you consume can make a drastic difference in your weight and the development of future illness. **Restricting carbohydrates, especially the bad ones, has proven to be the most effective diet.** Several studies have verified that weight loss on a low-carb diet was greater than on low-fat diets or those that blend fat and carbohydrate restrictions, like the Zone diet. In studies in which a traditional low-fat diet was compared to a carbohydrate-restricted diet, the low-carb one proved more successful for weight loss—and the weight was kept off after a year.

What this shows is that you should avoid sources of high glycemic loads, which, in Western civilization, are mostly bread, potatoes, sweetened soft drinks, candy, and desserts.

In Asia, the main offender is rice—which many Westerners think is so healthy. People who eat a lot of rice have a 75 percent increased risk of developing diabetes. (Chinese people have a diet that can be extremely high in carbohydrates; carbs often make up about 75 percent of their intake, which is around 300 grams of carbohydrates daily. American diets range closer to 200 grams.)

Lower Carbs, Better Results?

What are the metabolic effects of a low-carb diet? Will eating all of that fat, protein, and cholesterol have some type of ill effect on the body's cholesterol levels? Wasn't the low-fat diet originally recommended to have a more favorable effect on cholesterol?

Surprisingly, the results were even better than expected for research participants on a low-carbohydrate diet, even when they were following an Atkins-type of carbohydrate-restricted diet that emphasized meat, butter, and eggs. It turns out that the total cholesterol was not much affected by the carbohydrate-restricted diet; in fact, there were favorable changes in blood sugar, triglycerides, and good cholesterol—much better than on the low-fat diet. A low-carbohydrate, high-fat diet also lowered insulin levels and blood pressure more than its low-fat counterpart, but the differences were small (I have seen these results duplicated in my patients).

However, there are some problems with an Atkins-type diet. The food range is severely restricted and it is difficult for people to maintain for the long term. The diet also restricts nutrient-rich foods, like low glycemic fruits, vegetables, and grains, which have essential properties for long-term health. The final flaw with such blends of low-carbohydrate, low-fat diets is that they are potentially harmful for some people. Although the average person doesn't see much change in cholesterol, there are others who have dramatic rises in cholesterol levels on this type of diet; there is a hereditary difference in the way some people react to saturated fats and cholesterol. (I have seen occasional dangerous elevations of cholesterol on this type of meat, egg, and dairy-laden diet. If you choose to follow such a diet, I recommend you do it under medical supervision and that you closely monitor your cholesterol.)

I have had great success using a modification of the Atkins low-carbohydrate diet, which augments the variety of foods allowed and is far more nutritious. Furthermore, this Globe's Best Diet has a proven, long-term track record that not only promotes weight loss but also has favorable effects on disease development, such as cardiovascular diseases and cancer.

To sum up, a low-carbohydrate diet works better for weight loss than a low-fat diet and has a well-documented track record of favorable health effects. It is a proven success—and a better solution.

You have the power to make the right choices today. Make an affirmation that you will choose the foods that are good for your body. Reinforce that statement by substituting one healthy carbohydrate choice for one bad one—and continue that every day. Treat your body to the wonderful, natural, and nutritious foods that it wants and needs. Choose health, not disease.

Chapter 10: Introducing the Villain—Insulin

Insulin is an essential body enzyme released from the pancreas, and its function is to control excess sugar in the bloodstream and to protect the body from its harmful effects. To do that, insulin reduces blood sugar by storing it—predominantly in the form of fat. Insulin, therefore, is the enzyme of weight gain. There is no better way to gain weight than to get insulin involved.

You diabetics out there needn't panic: insulin is completely essential. In fact, we cannot live without it. Type I diabetes (mellitus) is caused by a complete lack of insulin, and it was a rapid and lethal disease until injectable insulin was discovered. But insulin is like anything else: some is good, but too much starts to have harmful effects.

I hear a lot of patients say, "Doc, I don't eat any sugar." By that, they mean they don't use table sugar (or sucrose) on their food or in their beverages. However, there is sugar in various forms in almost everything we eat. Some foods have natural sugar or fructose, which is present in fruits. There are also sugars in whole grain products, like bread and cereals, which are usually called maltose. Of course, many of the foods we eat have been processed, and the sugars in them have been highly concentrated (examples of this are cookies, candies, many breads, sodas, juices, cereals ... the list is too long to include them all, but most of these high-sugar items come in boxes or packages).

When these high-sugar foods are eaten, the body says, "There's too much sugar around. I need to send out insulin to bring the level down, but I'll save some of this sugar for later by making fat." The net result of this storage of calories is that you start to gain weight.

There is another downside to this process. Once your body brings the high sugar levels back down to a normal/borderline to low level, you start to get hungry again. you start to get hungry again! And it's pretty hard to lose weight when you're hungry all the time. Unfortunately, it takes only about two hours for your sugar levels to come down, which means if you eat a diet high in carbohydrates (especially if these are processed sugars), you will get hungry every two hours.

The process works like this: First you eat a high-sugar meal. Your body releases large amounts of insulin to control the sugar level. The excess sugar is stored as fat. As a result of insulin's action, the blood sugar is pounded lower. This low sugar level then stimulates hunger, making you crave another high-sugar meal. This process is repeated every few hours as your waistline expands. This happens every day, meal after meal. Add some sugar, add a little fat … add some more sugar, add some more fat. That's some diet!

Have you heard the old saying that two hours after eating Chinese food, you're hungry again? That's probably because you ate mostly rice, which is pure sugar.

Insulin and Illness

Insulin has other effects besides weight gain. It raises the triglyceride level in your body. Triglycerides are another type of fat transported in the blood. This is different from cholesterol, which is a building block for cell walls. The function of triglycerides is to serve as transport vehicles for excess energy in the system. Is it any surprise, then, that when insulin is activated by too much sugar, these sugar and energy transport vehicles are produced in massive quantities?

For a long time, it was debated whether triglycerides were harmful (in addition to cholesterol). It appears that the argument has finally been settled: triglycerides will mess up your coronary arteries. That's just what you need, isn't it? So we have another cycle now: sugar leading to triglyceride production then leading to messed-up coronary arteries.

Insulin also lowers your level of good cholesterol (which is the particle that removes bad cholesterol from your body and arteries and returns it to the liver for excretion). The lower your good cholesterol, the higher your risk of coronary artery disease.

Studies show that higher levels of insulin can cause a 40 percent greater risk of developing elevated blood pressure (hypertension). These high levels of insulin are strong predictors of future death from coronary heart disease.

The Low-Fat, High-Insulin Diet

You may have begun to wonder about this low-fat, high-carbohydrate diet you've been recommended to follow. All that sugar is going to raise your triglycerides, which will increase your odds of a heart attack. All that sugar will lower your good cholesterol, which will also raise your chance of a heart attack. Wasn't the point of a low-fat diet to *decrease* your chances of a heart attack? So isn't it producing contradictory results to what was intended? Yes, it is. That is why I'm writing this book.

The more concentrated sugars you eat, the more insulin you release and the fatter you get. Your good cholesterol and triglycerides also get affected at the same time. Your coronary arteries get messed up and your heart attack gets closer.

If you've been following your doctor's recommendations to cut down on your fat, then you've been trying hard to increase your non-fat food items (i.e., carbohydrates—a.k.a., sugar). As a result, your body has been having an insulin party. So is it any wonder that my patients had the audacity to get bigger and bigger on the diet that the medical profession recommended for losing weight?

The world is not flat—and the low-fat premise is wrong. We have been duped. The habits you have developed in the interest of health are the same ones making you fat and sick. You have to change the whole way you think about a healthy diet. In the next few chapters, I will guide you on a path toward lean health that is scientifically valid and tested. Don't experiment with your body any further in the low-fat lie.

Chapter 11: Momma and Popeye Were Right

Momma said, "Eat your vegetables if you want to grow up big and strong." She was 100 percent right! Popeye would always be on the verge of defeat before remembering his secret weapon: spinach. When he ate it, his strength and health would zoom to unimaginable levels. Thank God for Popeye, because if it hadn't been for him, I would never have touched a vegetable in my youth. It turns out that Popeye was right, too!

I know from my experience with many patients what you are probably thinking. I can almost see that scowl on your face. The truth is that most people do not like these wondrous gifts from Mother Nature. Many of you have made the decision in childhood that there are far better choices than vegetables when it comes to tasty foods. Now, I need you to reexamine that thought.

I also suffered from vegetable phobia. The mere mention of the word "vegetable" would cause me to cringe. As I progressed through medical school, I knew that I had to somehow make friends with these creatures, but I didn't know how.

Then I came across that seven-country study, which made it clear that vegetables were among the most important foods. The countries along the Mediterranean that have good weather and access to fresh vegetables are the healthiest. Those that are deprived of a warm climate and abundant agricultural gifts, like Finland, are plagued with early death. Yes, there is magic in a simple vegetable.

Further research has confirmed the magic. The DASH diet is

recommended to people who suffer from blood pressure problems. If the number of vegetable portions in the diet is increased, blood pressure drops. There have also been abundant studies to show other benefits of vegetables:

- Vegetables are linked to lower cases of stroke and cardiovascular diseases.

- Vegetables may protect against certain forms of cancer, such as mouth, stomach, and colorectal cancer. This is particularly true for nonstarchy vegetables like lettuce and for other leafy vegetables, such as bok choy, broccoli, garlic, and onions.

- Tomatoes may be particularly helpful for the prevention of prostate cancer in men. This is probably due to lycopene, which is responsible for the tomato's red hue.

- One recent report also showed that daily tomato intake resulted in a 13 percent reduction of bad cholesterol (LDL). It's a great tasting food that comes with great results.

- A diet high in green, leafy vegetables was found to lower cholesterol significantly.

- Most vegetables are high in natural fibers, which slow the absorption process and minimize insulin release. They also increase and prolong our sensation of fullness. So vegetables are a low-calorie food that provide fullness and nutrition, and minimize hunger. What's not to love?

- The dietary fiber in vegetables also helps promote bowel function, reduce constipation, and prevent the development of diverticular disease of the colon.

- Vegetables are low in fat and calories. No vegetable has cholesterol. They are the perfect diet food.

- Vegetables are high in potassium, and a high-potassium

diet lowers blood pressure and could decrease the risk of kidney stones and help prevent bone loss.

- High vegetable and fruit intake may reduce chances of diabetes.

- Vegetables and fruits protect your vision by guarding against cataracts and macular degeneration.

- Besides fiber, vegetables have massive amounts of other nutrients, including vitamins, minerals, and antioxidants—some even have large amounts of protein. You could survive strictly on these wonderful creatures if it weren't for their lack of vitamin B-12. Besides that, you could get everything you need in life from them. There are not too many foods that could boast that.

As John Lennon Said, Give Peas a Chance!

So why is the vegetable so misunderstood? My opinion is that some of it goes back to our childhood tastes. I have spoken with many patients who haven't given cauliflower or broccoli a chance in twenty years. They have developed a negative opinion about mushrooms, carrots, and celery and don't want to consider any other possibility. I am asking you to rethink your opinion and your tastes. Give vegetables another chance; in turn, they will give you another chance at good health.

Vegetables can provide some absolutely delightful meals. I invite you to try some of the fabulous recipes in the back of the book to embark on the road to enjoying the simple vegetable and a healthier way of eating. It is the same road toward weight loss success.

The Healthy Way to Veg Out

This is where it starts: in the supermarket. You cannot eat what you do not have! When you arrive at the supermarket, steer your cart directly to the fresh fruit and vegetable section and load up on one of everything. Retry all the different things that you rejected at a young age. I'm sure you will find a few friends that you had long ago abandoned.

Rediscover or perhaps try for the first time some of the many possibilities. The variety of what is available has improved with mass transit. When was the last time you tried bok choy, okra, watercress, or butternut squash?

Unlike potatoes, which are really a carbohydrate, sweet potatoes are delicious, lower in sugar, and are actually tastier than their white cousins. Carrots and celery make great portable snacks.

One overlooked item is the soybean. Most people in the United States don't appreciate it. Technically, the soybean is really a legume and products made from it, like tofu, are high in protein and beneficial oils. I was a reluctant convert to eating tofu, but you'll be surprised. The taste is very mild, so it absorbs the flavor of what is cooked with it. In that way, it is similar to mushrooms. So the soybean is definitely worth adding to your cart—and to your diet.

There are over fifty vegetables available in America—how many of them have you tried recently?

The next step after buying vegetables at the supermarket is coming home and actually cooking them! Try a few of my favorite recipes in the back of the book—and see what you have been missing out on all these years.

My mother was raised on a farm and had loved vegetables her whole life. She made a science out of deriving the greatest taste from the simplest foods. As I became willing, she shared these discoveries with me. I am sharing them with you now.

Among the recipes, I have some personal favorites. I love the garlic spinach. The roasted peppers are too sinfully good to seem healthy, but they are. I thank my wife for the killer salad, which is irreplaceable to me. Mom's cucumber salad is a delight. And the eggplant dishes are among my favorites. All of the many recipes in this book will allow you to do something good for yourself that actually *tastes* good.

Affirm to yourself that you will eat at least two vegetables a day. At first, that may seem like a lot, but it will become habit— and, soon, you will recognize this as one of the great pleasures in life. Healthy eating is joyous eating. It is about appreciating the many wonderful gifts that nature has provided and utilizing them to your maximum benefit for pleasure and for health.

Chapter 12: An Apple a Day is Bad for Business

There is good reason the Cretan diet, the healthiest in the world, is full of fruit. Fruit is one of nature's great gifts. Think about it: fruit trees just effortlessly present us with tasty and natural nutrition. There is no cultivation, plowing or tilling involved. What a wonderful thing! You don't have to slaughter a fruit tree; year after year, it gives you the gifts of health and pleasure.

Fruit is also an essential part of a lean, healthy body. Fruits' natural sugar, fructose, is beautifully presented in fiber-rich encasing. They are low glycemic index and load foods, which slows the absorption of sugar and prevents an insulin surge. As the fructose is slowly absorbed, it creates a long-lasting sensation of fullness or satiety and relief from hunger. There is no rebound hunger, like after a sugar fix.

In addition to having natural sugars and fiber, fruit is jam-packed with essential vitamins, minerals, antioxidants, and other nutrients. Nature has provided packets of life for our bodies! In fact, fruit is 80 percent water, just like we are. Fruit refreshes, rehydrates, and cleanses our bodies with fluids. It is also cholesterol free and most kinds are fat-free (avocados are an exception).

Fruit seems to have some protective effect against lung cancer. Chances of developing other cancers (such as those of the gastrointestinal and urinary systems) may also be decreased by adding more fruit to your diet.

There is building evidence that fruit improves mental awareness and memory, most likely because of their high vitamin B levels, and colorful fruit may have additional nutrient and health value. There has been speculation in the medical field for years that the colorful skins of fruit like blueberries, apples, and tomatoes have a magical chemical in them called flavonoids that could have outstanding effects. In fact, the seven-country study concluded that flavonoids predominantly present in fruit are largely responsible for lower rates of mortality—a fact that should have been more widely publicized. (I will discuss flavonoids more fully in a separate chapter, but for now suffice it to say that fruits have lots of them and they are very good for you.)

A Fruitful Diet

Fruits are wonderful snacks with a natural sweetness. For those of you who have poisoned your taste buds with processed foods like candies and sugar-loaded desserts, you may have forgotten the beauty of fruit. It may take some time to fully appreciate the sweetness that it has to offer.

In some ways, this is like quitting salt. Many people are addicted to heavily salting their food, so for the first few weeks that they don't use any, they feel that their food is tasteless. With time, their taste buds regain sensitivity and they become aware of many of the tastes that they had been unaware of for so long. The same is true in this case: once you stop poisoning your body with highly sugared foods, you will, with time, revere the taste of fruit.

The choices are limitless. I recommend you do the same exercise with fruit that I asked you to do with vegetables. Steer your cart directly to the fruit and vegetable section of your grocery store and retry all of the fruit that you have not tried in the last few years. In addition, more types of fruit have become available, routinely shipped in from Chile or other South American countries in the winter months. When I was a child, kiwi, passion fruit, and star fruit were unheard of. Now, many grocery stores offer them seasonally. There are opportunities year-round to enjoy a fantastic variety of fruit, so give these exotic ones a try. The diversity is amazing—not to mention the taste! Have you recently tried persimmons? Pomegranate? Papaya? Lychee? Guava? You won't regret it—and the benefits will be bountiful. The old standbys are wonderful, too. Don't forget to load up on all the berries, melons, plums, cherries, bananas, pineapples, grapefruits, grapes, tangerines, pears, and oranges that you can. All together, there are over forty kinds of fruit readily available in America. How many of these have you eaten recently?

For a real treat, put them all together. You will find a recipe for fruit salad in the back of this book. You can't get a simpler recipe, yet it is the highlight of my morning several days a week. Or treat yourself to a fruit salad for dessert!

Fruit should become a daily part of your nutrition routine. You should eat at least one portion in the morning as part of your breakfast, your whole breakfast, or a mid-morning snack.

Then you should add at least one other portion later in the day, as dessert after lunch or dinner. Fruit can also be a delicious snack between meals, or to fill your hunger later at night. For those who have a habit of snacking on junk food throughout the day or in the evening, a piece of fruit is a wonderful, healthy replacement to consider.

You should also try to make fruit a part of every meal, as well as eating it between meals. After all, the Cretans have it right; they eat a pound a day and live for a long time, loving it. Keep fruit in open view to encourage your family members to join in on healthy snacking instead of reaching for pantry items.

Fruit is essential to a healthy diet and helps you maintain a lean and healthy body. Incorporate it into your diet and your life by striving to eat at least two portions daily. Replace junk food snacks with healthy and delicious fruit, and repeat to yourself, "I am a healthy person and will demonstrate it in my choices and actions."

Chapter 13: The "Fats" of Life

Fat has gotten a bad name in our society. Everything is advertised as low fat or even nonfat. Everyone wants the fat out.

I have a problem with a fat-restricted diet. It teaches people to avoid and restrict fat at all costs. However, not all fat is bad. Nowhere in the Declaration of Independence does it say, "All fats are created equal." They are not.

Fats: The Good, the Bad, and the Lethal

Fats are an extremely diverse group, and their effects range from extremely dangerous to extremely beneficial. What would you say if I told you that one kind of fat lowers your risk of heart attack in half, but another kind more than doubles it? Would you restrict your fat intake? Well, if you've been doing what the medical profession has told you to do, then you have restricted fat—even though it is not entirely logical to restrict something that can cut your chances of a heart attack in half. In this way, fats are much like carbohydrates: selecting the right ones is absolutely critical for your health.

Does that mean we have to give up good taste? Absolutely not. Healthy fats can be just as appetizing and pleasurable as the lethal ones. In my opinion, the lethal fats taste nasty. If you make the right choice, you will not only improve your health but your taste also.

In general, fat intake can impact weight loss if done properly. Fat is much more slowly absorbed than carbohydrates and it does not cause an insulin surge like carbohydrates do. Fat usually takes three to four hours to be absorbed and, during that time, produces a sensation of fullness or satiety. There is no hypoglycemia and it does not cause rebound hunger a few hours later.

Therefore, careful ingestion of fat produces prolonged fullness that can contribute to weight loss. This has been verified on many occasions, particularly when nuts are used as a fat source. On the other hand, fat is very calorie rich, even more than carbohydrates. So you must exercise caution in terms of quantity. You can overdo fats like anything else, but the advantage is that they will minimize your hunger in a lasting way.

There are a few fats that are essential nutrients and are required for health, just like vitamins. There is also some evidence that a low-fat diet can produce osteoporosis, so some fat in the diet is optimal.

However, there is so much diversity among fats that it is best to break them down into separate chapters. We will start with the best, the omega-3 fats, then work our way down the chain to plant oils like olive and canola oil. We will then proceed to the more harmful saturated fats and finish with the lethal trans-fatty acid group.

By the time we're through, you will have learned all about "the fats of life"—which ones you should remove from your life altogether and which ones are essential to it.

Chapter 14: Amazing Omega-3 Fats—The Hidden Miracle

Would you like to lower your risk of heart attack dramatically? Would you like to do it while eating delicious and nutritious foods that promote lean health? Then omega-3 fats are for you. So where can you get this miraculous stuff?

Although omega-3 fats are considered essential nutrients, required for proper neurological functioning, they are not produced in the body. Instead, they are found predominantly in fish and nuts.

I imagine that some of you are groaning again because the mere thought of fish leaves a bad taste in your mouth. Most people have had a bad experience somewhere along the line that tainted their enjoyment of the healthiest food on earth. The same as with vegetables, however, it is time to give fish a second chance (I have some tricks ahead for those of you who find this task impossible).

The Benefits of Omega-3 Fats

It has been known for decades that Eskimos, who eat huge quantities of omega-3, have been miraculously protected from heart disease. They eat on average a half to one pound of omega-rich, fatty fish daily and experience only about one-fifth the number of heart attacks as the general population. The high intake of these omega-3s is also reflected in blood cholesterol levels that are 20 percent lower and triglyceride levels that are 60 percent lower than the total average.

The Japanese have also been beneficiaries of this miraculous compound. Although they eat about half the amount of omega-3s that Eskimos do (averaging one-quarter to a half pound of fatty fish daily), they are still greatly protected from coronary heart disease. Unfortunately, they eat about seven times the amount of omega-3 foods that Americans eat.

Medical science has added to this evidence. There have been a number of studies that observed the effects that fish or other omega-3 sources have had when added to the diet. The reports consistently show reduced heart attack rates (varying from 20 percent less in some studies to as much as seventy percent less in the Lyon heart study).

The Lyon heart study was landmark research in which patients were encouraged to eat a Cretan-like diet supplemented with omega-3 fats (although the Cretans eat huge amounts of fresh fruit and vegetables, they are not big fish eaters). The results were dramatic. It reduced heart attacks by 70 percent and patients lost weight. That's a home-run diet!

You may have been wondering how the Globe's Best Diet deviates from the Cretan or Mediterranean diet. I am recommending that you adopt their love of fresh vegetables and fruits but that you supplement this with fish and nuts. The Lyon heart study showed that if you add omega-3 to an already healthy diet, you get even better results. So the Globe's Best Diet combines some of the best eating (and best tasting) aspects of all cultures.

One Fish, Two Fish...

How much intake is required to start to see the benefits of omega-3? It doesn't take very much. Even small amounts of fish will do. In fact, one ounce daily will reduce coronary heart disease by half. The exact mechanism by which omega-3 fats lower cardiovascular risk is uncertain, but they do have a blood-thinning effect that could prevent clots in the arteries that cause heart attacks.

In a nurses' health study, there was an inverse relationship between fish intake and heart disease. They stratified the nurses into five groups, ranging from lowest to highest intake. Every time the intake of omega-3 was increased, the risk of heart problems was lowered. In the heavy fish-eating group, risk of heart attacks was half of what it was in the group that ate little or no fish. So even though a small amount will improve your health, when it comes to omega-3, the more, the better.

The positive effects that eating fish has on heart attack prevention have been well documented, but until recently it was unclear how well it prevented stroke. However, it turns out that it only takes eating fish a few times a month to reduce the risk of stroke in half. There is one exception: if you have had a hemorrhagic stroke, omega-3 (with its blood-thinning effects) may not be for you; there is a tendency for increased risk of stroke in this category.

In one study, people who ate fish only one to three times a month had fewer strokes (around 40 percent less). I think even those of you who don't like fish can accomplish that target.

Omega-3s also have beneficial effects on blood fats, specifically lowering triglycerides. As we saw earlier, triglycerides are elevated in obesity and cardio-metabolic syndrome, so it is extremely healthy to lower them naturally through high omega-3 intake.

These fats also raise good cholesterol (HDL). We discussed before how low good cholesterol is another part of cardio-metabolic syndrome, so this is helpful in its treatment. In fact, I recommend large quantities of omega-3 for all of my cardio-metabolic syndrome patients. There is no real downside to incorporating it into your diet.

Some studies also showed that as little as three grams of omega-3 daily lowered blood pressure by about five points. It has also had favorable effects on serum cholesterol, which may contribute to lower risk of cardiovascular disease, but it works predominantly through triglycerides and good cholesterol.

Omega-3 also has anti-inflammatory effects and can be helpful in some conditions that involve chronic pain and inflammation.

Breast cancer may be diminished by increased omega-3 intake. Even tumor growth in animals is suppressed by adding omega-3 to their diets.

All of these health benefits show that omega-3 fats are essential nutrients, like vitamins. The nerve tissue of the body needs a certain minimal amount of them to function properly. Have you ever heard that fish is brain food? Well, it's true. Omegas-3s are food for your brain and nerves.

For the majority of you reading this book, more is better when it comes to omega-3. There is no toxic dose. I've heard a few stories about fish contaminated with toxic minerals like mercury, but unless you are pregnant, there is no clinical significance to any such toxicity. I have never had a patient suffering from mercury poisoning by eating fish, but I have had thousands with cardio-metabolic syndrome, diabetes, coronary disease, high triglycerides, and all of the many conditions that benefit from the intake of omega-3.

Red Fish, Blue Fish?

Fortunately, there are many sources of omega-3, but I will start with the richest source, which is the fatty fish. Omega-3 in fact comes from the fat of fish. If you look at fish, you'll notice that some are round and fat, and others are flat. You want the round and fat kind. Below is a partial listing of fish sources of omega-3 and their relative contents. (Table 6)

Table 6: Omega-3 Rich Sources
Richest sources: salmon, tuna, halibut, trout, shark, anchovies, herring, kipper, pilchard, mackerel, sardines.

Medium content: rockfish, smelt, squid, swordfish, whitefish, turbot, sea bass.

Lower content: abalone, catfish, clams, crab, cod, flounder, grouper, haddock, lobster, mahi mahi, mussels, octopus, oysters, perch, pike, pollock, scallops, shrimp, snapper, sole.

Certainly if more is better, then focusing on the highest sources (like my favorites, trout and salmon) makes sense. On the other hand, it takes only small amounts of this miracle fat to see benefits, so there is no reason to snub even the weaker sources of omega-3.

However, there is one way you can mess up your omega-3 intake: in the preparation.

I recommend that you broil, poach, or steam your fish—or, if you are brave enough, eat your omega-3 sources raw (sushi or sashimi)! You may also try the fabulous recipes in the back of the book if you'd like to prepare your foods in great and healthy combinations. Make it a home run meal by adding vegetables and fruits to the mix (like the mango salmon, for example).

Frying fish can counteract and destroy some of its good effects. One study showed that people who ate fish sandwiches in fast food restaurants actually had higher incidences of cardiovascular problems! It is likely that the oils used to fry the fish had negative effects on the system. Therefore, if you must eat in a fast food restaurant, do not try to fool yourself into thinking that you are doing your body a favor with the fish sandwich. (I recommend staying away from these places altogether.)

Suppose, however, that you are either physically allergic or completely intolerant to eating fish? I have a few suggestions. The simplest one is to take fish oil capsules since even these small amounts can have beneficial effects on your arteries. I recommend that you get the one or one-and-a-half gram capsules of omega-3. (Some brands will just say "fish oil," some will say "salmon oil," or the label may just read "omega-3." It is not the brand that is important, but buying it and taking it!)

Even one of these capsules a day will provide you with some protection, not to mention essential nutrients. In a large European study, patients who took these supplements had fewer heart attacks and 14 percent fewer died prematurely. That is a pretty simple way to prolong your life.

If you are not a fish or nut eater, but are one of the many who suffer from diabetes, cardio-metabolic syndrome, or elevated triglycerides, then higher-dose omega-3 capsules are a good alternative. For people with triglycerides in the 200–300 range, two grams of fish oil with breakfast and dinner is a good dose; that is a total of four grams (or four capsules) daily. For those with triglycerides over 300 (as mine was when I first uncovered my cardio-metabolic syndrome), you should take a dose like I do, which is three grams of omega-3 with breakfast and dinner, or a total of six capsules daily.

These gel capsules resemble vitamin-E supplements and are not hard to take. However, some people feel they are too large to swallow comfortably, so they buy the liquid form at a vitamin store. Side effects are minimal. If you belch, you might get a fishy taste, but otherwise these supplements are free of negative consequences.

Some people don't take their fish oil on days when they have a large fatty fish intake, but that is up to the individual. With a daily dose of supplements, triglycerides commonly drop 40 percent or significantly higher. This is particularly true if you combine fish oil with a restriction of high glycemic carbohydrates. The results are phenomenal! I have actually cured cardio-metabolic syndrome with this type of diet.

Of course, another alternative to fish is to get your omega-3 from a different source, such as nuts (I will recommend other sources in later chapters). However, whichever source you use, you must incorporate omega-3 fats into your diet. They can promote lean health by filling you up with essential nutrients that prevent heart problems and untimely death. What more could you ask for?

Make the decision to add omega-3 as part of your daily lifestyle. Start today.

On your next trip to the market, load your cart with sources of omega-3 fats—it's like stocking up on a miracle! Eat fish or take fish oil—and make it a healthy habit. Your body will thank you for years to come.

Chapter 15: Nuts—the Secret Weight-Loss Weapon

Why nuts are such an unpopular snack is a mystery to me. I see and talk to very few nut eaters, and usually think of them as being a little unusual (I'm not saying that they're "nuts," just unusual!) Hopefully after you read this, you will become one of those unusual people yourself.

Most people think of nuts as fattening, which may be one reason for their lack of popularity. This could not be further from the truth, however. In fact, no other food has more evidence relating it to weight loss than the nut.

It is true that nuts are full of fat (which is why I'm including them in my section on fats and oils)—and if you've been listening to medical advice, you would avoid them on this fact alone. According to the old school of weight loss, if you avoid fatty foods that are calorie intense, you will lose weight; a low-fat diet is supposed to be good for health, and because nuts are full of fat, they must therefore be unhealthy. Isn't it interesting, then, that in an effort to lose weight people have been avoiding the one food that is most linked to weight loss?

People who consistently eat nuts *lose approximately seven pounds per year.* Add that to other interventions like exercise, careful carbohydrate selection, and augmentation of fruit and vegetable intake, and you are on the road to significant weight loss and a lean, healthy body.

"Good" Fat—In a Nutshell
There is an added benefit to nuts. The type of fat they have

is among the healthiest. Some nuts, especially walnuts, are high in omega-3 fats; the majority of fat in nuts is also healthy, monosaturated fat (which will be discussed later).

In my opinion, walnuts are the best of a very good group. As I said, they are extremely high in omega-3 and were found to lower cholesterol and triglycerides. I am such a big fan of walnuts that I buy a large bag every week and keep it on my desk for between-meals snacks. They are delicious and very popular with visitors to my office. If you are the kind of person who finds yourself visiting the candy machine mid-morning or mid-afternoon, then nuts are a great solution to your problem. You will replace empty sugar calories that promote weight gain with artery-cleaning, life-prolonging, delicious food.

All nuts suppress hunger for prolonged periods because of their high-fat constitution, but many of them have even been studied individually. Almonds were found to lower cholesterol and are part of the DART diet for blood pressure reduction. Macadamia nuts are so delicious that they are addicting; they are also extremely high in healthy, monosaturated fats and have been found to lower cholesterol (their only drawback is expense, but for an occasional treat they can't be beat). There have also been studies on pistachios and pecans that have confirmed their beneficial effects. For those of you who simply can't stand nuts, flaxseed is another related plant origin high in omega-3.

The physicians' health study showed that the more nuts people ate, the less their chances of dying (due to the benefits of omega-3). Nuts, including peanut butter, decrease your cholesterol (particularly the bad, LDL type) by about 10 percent, and people who consume nuts daily lower their chances of developing diabetes by 27 percent. This result is possibly due to the weight loss or because this healthy food was substituted for high glycemic index foods, thus lowering their risk of disease.

The addition of nuts is just another way that the Globe's Best Diet differs from the typical Mediterranean diet. If you refer to Table 4, page 63, you will see that nuts are not a large component of what is considered the typical Cretan diet. The traditional Cretan diet is rich in olive oil, but a recent study showed that substituting nuts for olive oil resulted in reducing cardio-metabolic syndrome in half. Both the olive oil and the nut supplemented Mediterranean diets were far better for preventing cardio-metabolic syndrome than the typical low fat diet. The nut supplemented diet decreasing cardio-metabolic syndrome by 70 percent! For those that were able to maintain this diet long term, the results were even more dramatic. A low fat diet was six times as likely to lead to cardio-metabolic syndrome than a Mediterranean diet supplemented with nuts.

In any case, the benefits of nuts are multiple. They are a delicious food, a healthy snack, a perfect substitute for high glycemic index foods, and a way to prolong and enhance your life. Eating nuts promotes weight loss, lowers cholesterol and triglycerides, and prevents diabetes and death! Why would you not make something like this a part of your daily routine?

In fact, start today. After you steer your cart to the fruit and vegetable section of the supermarket, go straight to the nut section and load up on the many wonderful, healthy choices. Mixed nuts are an especially good way to get a tremendous variety of tastes.

Make this a regular part of your shopping trip and daily routine. Bring nuts to work and substitute them for other unhealthy snacks. When coworkers offer you junk food, reply, "No, thanks, I have something better. Would you like some?" (I'm telling you, walnuts do the trick!)

Also, make an affirmation to lose weight the delicious and healthy way by eating natural nuts instead of the sugary snack foods that you've been poisoning your body with. You'd have to be nuts *not* to!

Chapter 16: Cooking and Salad Oils

What oil you use to cook and make your salad dressing may not affect your weight much, but your life may depend on it! There are major differences in the outcomes of our health that can be attributed to kitchen habits. I highlighted this earlier when I said that fish was extremely healthy as long as it wasn't fried. Similarly, it is likely that certain cooking oils can cause some serious risk to otherwise healthy food. If you're making this mistake at home, you can turn all of your meals into a future heart attack.

A good part of the reason Cretans have such few heart attacks is their choice of oil. They almost exclusively use olive oil in their cooking and salads. Olive trees are plentiful there, and it is just a matter of using what you have that tastes good.

The benefits of this oil have been verified in other populations. In one study, people who exclusively used olive oil in daily cooking and food preparation were shown to have 47 percent fewer heart problems. That is a pretty simple change that produces dramatic results.

Olive oil has other benefits as well. It has predominantly monosaturated fat. It is chemically easy on the system. It lowers blood cholesterol and improves blood sugar.

It is a slowly absorbed fat that promotes prolonged satiety. It has been documented to lower insulin levels, decreasing weight gain and the development of cardio-metabolic syndrome.

With such a track record overall, you'd have to ask yourself why you'd use anything else. The answer is that you may possibly be able to do even better.

There are cooking oils that also contain the magical omega-3 fats. Of these, my favorite is canola oil, which has 30 percent omega-3 and 54 percent monosaturated fat. As we've seen, omega-3 has beneficial effects on good (HDL) cholesterol and triglycerides, and monosaturated fats lower bad cholesterol. This particular win-win combination was the one used in the Lyon heart study that advised a Cretan-like diet modified by an addition of oils rich in omega-3. With that dietary combination, patients had a 70 percent reduction in cardiovascular events.

Although the jury is still out as to which one is better, I lean toward the canola camp, but believe that you cannot go wrong with olive oil, either. There are some other oils that also deserve honorable mention. Soybean and flax both have high amounts of omega-3 and monosaturated fats. In fact, soybean oil may be responsible for the low rates of heart problems in the Japanese population (therefore, I have included soy recipes as part of the internationally influenced Globe's Best Diet). Flax was associated with protection from heart disease in the nurses' health study.

Don't Be Fooled by "Snake Oil"

These four oils—olive, canola, flax, and soybean—complete the recommended category. However, many of you may still be waiting for me to mention the oil you use … and you may see it now, in the less desirable category that includes corn, safflower, sunflower, sesame, cottonseed, and peanut oils.

Early in medical history, there was a theory that plant origins were good and animal origins were bad. This mostly came from the seven-country study that found that animal fats were linked to heart disease. While it is true that some plant oils do lower cholesterol (in some cases, better than monosaturated fats like olive oil), there is also a downside. For one thing, they lower good cholesterol.

Another adverse effect of these oils is that they compete with the miraculous omega-3 and can counterbalance many of its good effects. As a result, I do not recommend these oils. Buy and exclusively use the big four listed above.

Now, let's move on from the less desirable oils to the downright dangerous ones. If you have any of these oils in your refrigerator, I want you to walk over and throw them out right now: coconut oil, palm oil, butter, and lard. These are laden with dangerous, saturated fat. It is one thing to occasionally nibble on some nutritious foods like dairy products and meats that have saturated fat as components of their nutrition, but it is simply bad judgment to add saturated fat without any other nutritional benefit to all of your cooking. It's like sprinkling a little artery killer and death into your food.

The choice is simple and straightforward. You need to buy and use only the right kinds of oil. If you make the wrong choice, the consequences are lethal.

Make the decision to substitute healthy oils for dangerous ones and empty your refrigerators and pantries of bad choices. On your next trip to the store, buy only olive, canola, soybean, or flax oil—and always use it. It's amazing that Americans are more careful about which types of oil they put in their cars than in their bodies! Accept no substitutes when it comes to your health, and avoid well-advertised "snake oils" at all costs.

Chapter 17: Hidden Poisons in Your Diet and the Trans-Fatty Acid Lies

The trans-fatty acid story is so horrific that I'm surprised it hasn't been on *60 Minutes* or made into a horror film like *The Blob*. It's the tale of good medical science gone loco and the food industry's shameless promotion of this poison. And it's a story that ends with approximately thirty thousand premature deaths every year. A whiff of this poison will increase your chances of a heart attack by 50 percent—and you eat it every day without even knowing it.

The trans-fatty acid scandal started after the seven-country study, which showed that a low intake of saturated fat like that derived from dairy and animals was most desirable, and that a high intake of vegetable products was preferred.

At that time, America was an egg with buttered toast kind of population (butter is a dairy product with saturated fat). Then medical science came up with an alternative to butter, using a vegetable oil instead. This in itself would have been a decent idea, but they decided to market it in a way that was spreadable, which is where the story, I think, goes awry. The food industry found that if they processed the vegetable oil, they could make it solid (by this point in the book, you should already be hearing bells go off when you see the word "processed"). The process is called "partial hydrogenation." Remember those words as ones you never want to see on any label.

What do you call a healthy vegetable oil that has been processed and changed into a harmful chemical? You call this product margarine. In the interest of health, Americans were asked to give up their delicious butter and change to less palatable, lethal margarine—and millions of people did. The result was that they got sicker than they ever would have if they had stuck with natural butter.

Here are the reasons: The body is not prepared to handle chemically altered, unnatural foods. They produce unexpected ill effects on the system. For instance, margarine is worse for your cholesterol system than butter, the natural product it was meant to replace. It raises bad (LDL) cholesterol significantly, just like butter, but also dramatically lowers good (HDL) cholesterol, unlike butter. Margarine also raises triglycerides. This is a terrible combination. To raise bad and lower good cholesterol makes the ratio of bad to good really high. There could not be a worse formula for artery health, yet this is what was recommended—especially for those who had heart problems! (I can remember recommending this poison to heart patients myself before I became enlightened around 2000.)

The effects of such processed food on the cardiovascular system are just what you would expect. There is a 40 percent rise in cardiovascular risk in people who ingest this poison!

Again, isn't it ironic that the very people who need the best medical care (heart patients) are advised to eat what is the worst possible and most immediately dangerous food for them?

Trans-fatty acids also affect the body's ability to handle sugars. The result can be higher insulin levels and the development of cardio-metabolic syndrome and weight gain.

The Poison You Are Putting in Your Mouth

So, how much of this stuff do you eat, anyway? The average daily intake is eight to ten grams or about 6 to 8 percent of your total daily fat consumption. It doesn't take very much of this poison to do damage. It is thought that if only 3 percent of your food intake is comprised of trans-fatty acids, your risk of cardiovascular disease will increase by 50 percent.

And where, exactly, do you find this stuff so you can avoid

it? Unfortunately, it is a secret. For many years, there was no requirement to quantify the amount of trans-fatty acids in foods. Luckily, those rules are beginning to change. The biggest clue that you shouldn't be eating something is if the label includes partially hydrogenated anything. The oil that follows, usually soybean or peanut, has been chemically processed to speed up your death. *Do not eat foods that have been partially hydrogenated or that have trans-fatty acids in them!*

The main offenders you'll find in supermarkets are as follows in Table 7.

Table 7: Trans Fatty Acid Sources
Food Grams of Trans-Fatty Acids / Serving

Margarine: 25
Microwave popcorn: 12
Potato chips: 10
Cracker: 8
Taco shell: 8
Glazed doughnut: 6
Chocolate chip cookie: 6
Pound cake: 5
French fries: 5
Vanilla wafer: 4
Tortilla chips: 4
Biscuit: 4
Chocolate: 3

One doughnut at breakfast and french fries at lunch will add eleven grams of trans-fatty acids to your diet, making your eighteen hundred calorie consumption composed of 5 percent trans-fatty acid. That's enough to drastically increase your chances of a heart attack or heart bypass. A doughnut a day does not keep the doctor away. A doughnut a day is good for our business.

If you can't eat margarine and you shouldn't eat butter, either, then what do you eat?

On bread, the Italians and Greeks use olive oil (you may have seen this in restaurants); sometimes, Italian seasoning is added for flavor. There are also some brands of margarine that are trans-free. If you can't use olive oil then consider using Promise margarine or tubs of Fleishmann's made from canola oil.

Many trans-fatty foods can be easily avoided if you bypass the entire nonrefrigerated center aisles in the supermarket, where the majority of packaged and processed foods are kept. Crossing those off your grocery list forever will help you to avoid a great portion of these villainous foods. If you stick to the periphery of the supermarket, where the fresh fruits and vegetables and refrigerated fish and meats are, you will zoom in on the nutritious food that lacks these dangerous chemicals. When in doubt, read the label and look for partially hydrogenated ingredients.

There is a reason these trans-fatty acid foods can sit unrefrigerated on store shelves and in machines. Have you ever wondered why they don't spoil? The chemicals used in processing are so toxic that many of the organisms involved in the decaying process cannot digest them. They are poisonous to those organisms, just as they are poisonous to you.

So now you know how to navigate around them in a supermarket. But what if the food is not labeled because it comes from a fast food restaurant? How do you know if there are trans-fatty acids in what you're eating?

You don't know for sure—but there probably is! Fast food restaurants are trans-fatty acid hell. They cook food in liquid death. Why? Because we asked them to! When all of the scientific research about the effects of animal fat was released, there was a public outcry to stop fast food chains, especially "the golden arches," from cooking with beef tallow. When they switched, they chose inexpensive trans-fatty acids as the alternative. We asked for vegetable fat, and we got it—only the vegetable fat has been chemically modified to speed up the hardening of the arteries more than beef tallow.

Just so you know what you're getting, some fast food trans-fatty acid contents are listed here in Table 8:.

Table 8: Trans-fatty Acid Content of Fast Foods

Trans-fatty Acid Content of Fast Food (grams/serving)
Long John Silver fish: 14
Burger King french fries: 7
Cinnabon: 6
McDonald's french fries: 4
KFC biscuit: 4
Burger King fish sandwich: 3
McDonald's chicken nuggets: 2
Burger King chicken sandwich: 2

As I mentioned earlier, if you eat a fried fish sandwich in a fast food restaurant, you are not doing yourself any favors health-wise. You more than counterbalance the good effects of omega-3 with the trans-fatty acids you are ingesting.

With so much fast food being tarnished with these poisons, you would be best to avoid such places altogether. People who successfully lost weight averaged just one visit a week to a fast food restaurant; instead, many of them used liquid meal replacements for lunch in addition to some of the healthy alternatives I have discussed. Although I have no affiliation with any of the chains, there are some that may offer healthier choices (for example, Boston Market sells rotisserie chicken and a good variety of vegetables for a healthier lunch choice).

Anything fried is suspect. Unless you were there during the frying process, you have no way of knowing what you are eating—and there is a good chance that you are inadvertently ingesting poisonous materials. If you must eat fried foods, it is safer to do so at home where you can control the ingredients. Ideally, you would use olive or canola oil.

As you might expect, the Greek diet originally documented in the seven-country study is extremely low in trans-fatty acids. Unfortunately, patterns change over time and with "progress," and the Cretans are not as limited now as they were in the 1950s through 1970s. However, they are moving in the wrong direction toward more trans-fatty foods.

Other countries (like France, for example) have low trans-fatty acid intake, and some people see this as a partial basis for the French paradox, explaining how the French can have a diet fairly high in fat (particularly butter), yet not have very much cardiovascular disease. It is possible that the type of fat consumed is more important than the quantity, and their diet is particularly low in the dangerous trans-fatty forms.

A Change Will Do You Good

It really doesn't take much change to improve your health risks by decreasing your trans-fatty acid intake. If you were to replace just 2 percent of your daily calories from trans-fatty acids to foods that are high in beneficial fats like omega-3 or healthy table oils, you could reduce your cardiovascular risk by 50 percent.

The bottom line is this: If you have any concern for your health at all and are not interested in multiplying your risk of heart attack, stay away from these dangerous chemicals and stick with natural, healthy, delicious, and unprocessed foods. Make a decision to avoid these processed poisons at every turn and choose healthier alternatives by avoiding the center aisles in the supermarket.

Plan ahead for lunch and avoid liquid death whenever possible. Bring along fresh fruit and nuts for snacks. Throw away your margarine and use healthier alternatives. Microwave fresh popcorn and avoid prepackaged chemicals. Just say no to artery death.

Chapter 18: Saturated Fats

Unless you've been living away from any news media (and I can't imagine where on earth that would be anymore), you have heard by now that saturated fats increase your chances of heart and other cardiovascular diseases. You have probably also heard that they raise bad cholesterol. But is it really true?

If the seven-country study showed one thing, it is that saturated fat is harmful to the human body. It is clear that the higher the intake, the higher the risk of cardiovascular disease. This single fact is the basis for all of the low-fat brainwashing that has infiltrated our society.

Saturated fat accomplishes its ill effects by raising both your cholesterol and triglycerides, which is probably how the risk of heart disease is increased. Moreover, saturated fats are associated with insulin resistance, meaning they promote more insulin release and, with it, the development of obesity and cardio-metabolic syndrome.

Focus on the Right Fats

It is wise to limit your consumption of foods high in saturated fats—but not all meat and dairy products are equal when it comes to intake. Table 9 below will show you which foods are the main culprits for saturated fat:

Table 9: Saturated Fat Content of Foods

Grams of Saturated Fat / 100 Grams of Food

Meats
Lard: 42
Salami: 18
Bacon: 17
Sausage: 14
Lamb chop: 11
Hot dog: 10
Sirloin roast: 9
Turkey: 9
Hamburger: 7
Duck: 3
Chicken: 2

Dairy
Butter: 49
Cheddar cheese: 20
Cheesecake: 19
Chocolate square: 18
Blue cheese: 17
Scrambled egg with cheese: 11
Pizza: 5
Cheese omelet: 5
Macaroni and cheese: 5
Ice cream: 4
Cottage cheese: 2
Whole milk: 2
Skim milk: 0.4
Swiss cheese: 0

Miscellaneous
French dressing: 10

Peanut butter: 10
Fruits: 0
Vegetables: 0

It is no surprise that processed meats fared the worst. Bacon, salami, sausage, and hot dogs head the list of saturated fat content. It is also no shock that the wrong cooking oils, like lard and butter, have ridiculously high contents.

Chicken, duck, and low-fat dairy products have negligible amounts of saturated fats compared to red meats, processed meats, and the bad cooking oils. Most people think of red meat as bad, unaware that processed meats are far worse, and they avoid even low-fat dairy products, although these provide calcium and vitamin D but contain only small amounts of saturated fats.

You certainly do want to keep your red meats to a minimum, however, so here are a few tips for reducing fat in the meat you eat:

- Instead of making meat the focus of your meal, make the vegetables your main focus. Prepare dishes that are full of vegetables and are accented with meat. Examples are stir fries, stews, and casseroles (consult the recipe list in the back).

- Trim the fat and buy meats that are less marbled.

- Choose the leanest meats; these are labeled "select" as opposed to "choice" or "prime."

- Eat game meats like venison and rabbit when available since they are lower in fat.

- Broiling will remove fat via dripping—unlike frying, which will add fat. Choose broiling over frying in food preparation.

Dairy and meat products are the main sources of saturated fats and should be selected cautiously and eaten in moderation (for example, low-fat dairy products, Swiss cheese, cottage cheese, chicken, and duck are reasonably low in saturated fats). However, the good news is that these foods do provide fullness. They are slowly absorbed and do not stimulate insulin—factors that make them more effective for weight loss than carbohydrates.

Also, for the majority of people, the effects of saturated fat on blood cholesterol are exaggerated, especially since blood cholesterol is predominantly controlled by genetic factors. Many patients debate daily whether they should eat a single slice of cheese, believing that having that one slice will shove their cholesterol reading up fifty points or avoiding it will lower their reading by fifty points. Most people's blood cholesterol will change only a point or so over these types of small decisions. If you really want a drop of thirty or more points, seriously consider taking medicine and stop struggling over a slice of cheese or an occasional steak. Your enjoyment of life will improve, along with your numbers.

When I was following a low-fat diet, I would beat myself up every time I had a steak, dairy product, or slice of cheese—until I finally realized that my numbers had never improved once during ten years of fat restriction. So I opted for cholesterol medication and abandoned the low-fat fight. The result? My cholesterol reading is now the best it has ever been. Sure, I eat lots of omega-3 fats, nuts, vegetables, and fruits—but I also eat steak and dairy on occasion when I feel like it without all the guilt I had on the low-fat diet.

Eliminate All Fats? Fat Chance!

I've seen the same results repeated hundreds of times in my patients who agonize over every deviation from their low-fat diets. If a person changes from a heavy meat and dairy diet to severe restriction, there is occasionally a twenty to thirty point drop in cholesterol, but most people already moderate their intake and do not eat steak and ice cream on a daily basis. For them, minor changes produce minor and disappointing results in blood cholesterol.

Studies confirm that people on Atkins-type diets, which are heavy in cream and meats, for the large part show no or only minor and insignificant changes in cholesterol. Diets like these, without extensive vegetable and fruit intake, are quite similar to the Finnish and American diets of the 1950s that were associated with a high heart attack rate. The fats may increase cardiac risk through other ways than just raising cholesterol and the long-term effects of such diets may be dangerous.

There are also some patients who are quite sensitive to saturated fats and their cholesterol will explode through the roof with very high intake. That is why I cannot fully endorse Atkins-style carbohydrate-restricted diets. The concept of limiting carbohydrates—especially processed and packaged, high glycemic ones—is entirely sound. The Atkins diet, however, substitutes large quantities of saturated fat foods for these wasteful carbohydrates, but also for some of the healthy carbohydrate choices.

I prefer a substitution of more favorable fats, like omega-3 and monosaturated fats, to the high-saturated fat intake of Atkins. I also recommend preserving the nutritionally charged carbohydrates contained in fruits and vegetables to promote long-term health, which Atkins does not. It makes sense to me that the moderate intake of select saturated fats can provide more nutrition than snacks with empty carbohydrates. In other words, if you have a beef and vegetable stir fry, you will get more nutrition and experience less weight gain than by eating a large bowl of pasta. Or if you have some whole grain cereal with low-fat milk, the benefits would be greater than those from eating a stack of pancakes with syrup.

These are all second and third choices, however. If you have maximized your fruit, vegetable, nut, and fish intake for the day, then a saturated fat alternative could be a better choice than a pure sugar meal. But if your choice is a fruit bowl or a pile of bacon, you should choose the fruit bowl every time.

Recently, the medical world has become aware of extremely frequent vitamin D deficiencies in adults, which have contributed to a more common diagnosis of osteoporosis. It is likely that the avoidance of dairy fat over the last thirty years has added to this epidemic. Therefore, occasional dairy products are of some benefit to your diet.

As you can see, saturated fats have contradictory effects on the system. They are not nutritionally empty, like processed carbohydrates, and most of them come with associated protein, vitamin D, or calcium. On the other hand, they promote hardening of the arteries, have lots of calories, and if not moderated will produce weight gain. If eaten in moderation, though, they do provide long-term fullness without stimulating insulin.

In conclusion, you should add fats to your diet, particularly those sources rich in omega-3, like fish, nuts, and the healthier olive and canola oils. If you restrict your fats, continue with meat and dairy in moderation, but do not expect major cholesterol improvement. Augment your fruits and vegetables to minimize your saturated fat intake, and combine them with meat dishes, such as many of those suggested in the recipe section.

Make a decision to select the right fats as often as possible and avoid the unhealthy ones (what I call the "fatal fats"). Start in the supermarket by filling your cart first with healthy fruits, vegetables, and nuts, and try to plan a few meals a week that focus on omega-3 fatty sources, like fish. Lastly, add carefully chosen meat and dairy selections and avoid processed meats, butter, and lard. Combine your well-thought-out meat and dairy choices with healthier alternatives to make a balanced meal. Careful use of these foods can add nutrition and prevent the weight gain associated with America's sugar habit.

You can make better choices when it comes to saturated fats—starting with your next meal—and limit the quantity and frequency of less healthy fat sources. In this way, you'll free yourself of the guilt associated with deviating from the low-fat lifestyle. Not only will you feel healthier, you may also enjoy your meals more!

Chapter 19: The New Hero—Flavonoids

Flavonoids are the secret miracle in medicine—so secret that most people have never heard of them. One of the major conclusions of the seven-country study was to eat more flavonoids in order to protect against cardiovascular disease. In spite of that, however, they remain largely anonymous. Flavonoids definitely need a better press agent! In the meantime, allow me to introduce them to you now.

Flavonoids are powerful antioxidants present in many natural foods that help protect the arteries from the damaging effects of cholesterol and oxygen working together. There are over four thousand varieties of flavonoids identified in various plants. You can usually see them because they are responsible for the bright external covering on many fruits and vegetables. The brilliant hues of tomatoes, apples, oranges, and blueberries, as well as the deep, dark color of cocoa, are all due to flavonoid components. Other major sources, in addition to fruits and vegetables, are tea, wine, and juices.

There is significant data linking flavonoid consumption to protection from cancers of the breast, urinary tract, gastrointestinal tract, and lungs. Numerous studies have also linked high intake of flavonoids to reduced risk of death from cardiovascular disease by about 50 percent.

Flavor Flavs

The benefits of flavonoids are serious—but eating healthy can be fun. One of the most potent sources of flavonoids as antioxidants is chocolate derived from the cocoa plant. In Woody Allen's movie *Sleeper*, the main character awakens in the future to find out that the healthiest food has been discovered to be chocolate ice cream. I'm not sure about the ice cream part but as far as chocolate is concerned, the future is here!

It's obvious that medicine can throw us some strange curves when something as good as chocolate is also found to be healthy. But not just any chocolate will do—it has to be dark chocolate, probably because the rich color points to the increased presence of flavonoids.

This is not an open invitation to eat as much chocolate as you'd like, however. Some flavonoids are in fact destroyed in the chocolate-making process; therefore, candy bars are less rich in flavonoids than are purer sources. The problem is that flavonoids do not appear on food labels, so there is no guarantee of content. A good guideline is to go for the dark pieces with higher cocoa percentages.

People who eat small amounts of chocolate daily (about five grams, or one-sixth of an ounce) can expect to see their blood pressure reduced by nearly three to four points—plus, they will not gain weight with this small amount. As we saw earlier, chocolate has a lot of saturated fat, so large amounts will cause weight gain or have adverse effects on cholesterol.

In longer-term studies, people who ate the right amount of chocolate were about 50 percent less likely to die from any cause! It's unbelievable that eating chocolate decreases your chances of dying by half but, happily, it's true.

Tea Time

Green and black teas are also rich sources of flavonoids. These delicious beverages are not as popular in America as coffee is, but they are significantly healthier. Regular coffee doesn't have as many flavonoids as green tea—still; it is not as risky as the decaf version, which is associated with a 25 percent increase in the risk of heart attacks.

The Japanese have it right. Tea is responsible for 80 percent of their flavonoid intake. They are especially big drinkers of green tea, which may be partially responsible for their low rates of cardiovascular disease. Both green and black teas are derived from the leaves of *camellia sinensis*; while green tea is high in the flavonoid called catechin, black tea is high in the one known as theaflavin—and both have beneficial health effects.

In a study of Japanese patients, it was shown that green tea had life-preserving capabilities. These active flavonoids, studied in capsule form, lowered bad (LDL) cholesterol by about 16 percent and triglycerides by 11 percent (most people just drink the tea, however, and forgo the capsule extracts). Higher green tea intake also correlates with lower mortality. This was evident even with one to two cups daily—but the more, the better. The maximum benefit was seen in those who drank five cups or more a day and were able to lower their mortality risk by 17 percent. Another study concluded that tea drinkers reduce their chances of heart attacks by 44 percent. So there are times when living a healthy lifestyle can provide great enjoyment—and refreshment, too.

The Cretan diet is not particularly high in cocoa, nor is it high in other flavonoid choices like tea. However, it is rich in fruit and vegetable sources, so a combination of both is another example of how the Globe's Best Diet works by providing the ultimate food and nutrition choices culled from around the globe.

Don't Just Whine About Eating Healthy—Drink Wine!

In Greece, the main sources of flavonoids are apples and onions—and if you cook with these, you not only add flavor but life-preserving flavonoids to your meals. The United States also commonly utilizes these rich sources of flavonoids but our intake is nowhere near what it is in the more rural areas of Greece.

There is good news, though. Another rich source of flavonoids (particularly quercetin and catechin) is wine, especially red wine in the varietals of pinot noir, merlot, and cabernet sauvignon (white chardonnay also has a fair number of flavonoids). This rich source, enjoyed throughout France and Italy, is thought to be another possible explanation for the French paradox, balancing out their high-fat diets.

One study showed that light drinkers of wine had a 30 percent reduction in mortality compared to only a 10 percent reduction in light drinkers of other alcoholic beverages. This may be further evidence of the magical effects of flavonoids, more so than the effects of the alcohol itself. (Other studies show similar trends, but to a less dramatic degree.) The theory goes that one to two glasses of red wine daily contain enough flavonoids to provide protection. Flavonoids may also increase the health of the neurological system, in addition to their vascular effects. French people who drank three glasses of wine daily had a 75 percent reduction in Alzheimer's disease. So flavonoids are absolute magic for the vessels and the brain.

To all you beer drinkers out there: sorry, but because beer is derived from hops and barley, not colorful grapes, it is generally low in protective flavonoids, as are other alcoholic spirits. An exception may be dark beer, which seems to offer some protective results. The dark color points to the presence of flavonoids (in this case, quercetin, reservatrol, and rutin, all of which have antioxidant effects).

Again, this is not a license to drink as much wine or dark beer as possible before passing out (you'll see my warnings regarding alcohol use in the next chapter). And if you are at risk for alcoholism and have to abstain from the benefits of red wine, I have another suggestion. It turns out that purple grape juice has many of the same beneficial flavonoids without the risky alcohol intake. A small amount is all that is needed, approximately four to eight ounces daily. Purple grape juice has been documented to have favorable results on the circulatory system and provide some blood thinning effects, like aspirin, so there is a two-for-one benefit.

Grapes themselves, however, do not fare as well. The amount

of flavonoids in these fruits differs greatly among grape varieties: purple grapes in general tend to be higher in flavonoids, but the specific varietals used to make wine are much better than store-bought varieties. Their beneficial effects are concentrated in the juice and wine.

Other fruit juices may also provide protection. Consumption of fruit or vegetable juice three times weekly decreases the risk of Alzheimer's disease by as much as 75 percent (the same as red wine). Especially powerful is apple juice, which is particularly high in the potent flavonoid quercetin.

A Grocery List of Life's Pleasures
In Table 10 are some selected foods and their flavonoid levels:

Table 10: Selected Flavonoid-Rich Foods

Low (<10 mg/kg): cabbage, carrot, mushroom, pea, spinach, peach, white wine, coffee, orange juice

Medium (<50mg/kg): lettuce, tomato, red pepper, broad bean, strawberry, apple, grape, red wine, tea, tomato juice

High (>50 mg/kg): onion, kale, French bean, broccoli, endive, celery, cranberry.

Now that you know what flavonoids are, you have to admit that eating them is tasty and just plain fun. A small piece of dark chocolate, a glass of red wine, and a cup of delicious green tea are just some of life's pleasures that provide good health and good taste all in one. Think of them as "guilty pleasures" that you can enjoy every day—only without the guilt!

Chapter 20: Alcohol—the Two-Faced Friend

"Alcohol can save your life." "Alcohol can kill you and destroy your life." Which of these statements is true depends on you and your makeup. I know because I have lived on both sides of the fence.

Alcohol-related deaths have been estimated at one hundred thousand annually. On the other side of the coin, if everyone became a non-drinker, heart disease-related deaths would increase by eighty thousand a year. Maybe it comes down to simple math: if you are in the category of having four or more drinks daily, then the odds are good that you *increase* rather than decrease your chance of dying.

So I will start with the warnings first: alcohol is cunning, baffling and powerful. It can cause addiction, which can start the process of denial. The mind will use any excuse to continue drinking despite significant evidence that it is ruining your life. Cloudy judgment will struggle to justify, at all costs, that alcohol is not the problem.

It is for this reason that I cannot give a blanket recommendation to consume alcohol. There are some people who will be destroyed if they follow that path. How do you know if you are one of them? There are classic signs: if you have memory blackouts, get arrested for DUI, need alcohol in the morning to open your eyes, or have the shakes when you don't drink, then it is obvious. If there is a family history of alcoholism then maybe you shouldn't even attempt to add alcohol to your dietary program.

I'd also like to add some subtler signs that may tip you off about whether or not you need treatment or should guard against alcohol use. If you look forward to any ethnic holidays that do not pertain to you (such as St. Patrick's Day, Cinco de Mayo or, in some cases, even New Year's) simply because they are occasions for drinking, then beware. If you cannot imagine a holiday with relatives *without* imbibing alcohol, you may have a problem. If all of your activities are centered on alcohol, then there is a *definite* problem. If you look to alcohol as a solution when you have emotional stress, then that is a red flag. If you must take every good occasion to the next level through the use of alcohol in order to feel that you are really celebrating, then be careful. And if you are the kind of person who can never have one drink or leave a glass half empty, then that is an indication of a serious issue.

Too Much of a Good Thing

Having made all those warnings, let me state that alcohol in moderation can definitely provide some benefit to your heart. The key is *moderation*. For women, that means one drink daily (maybe two if you are larger). For men, one to four drinks daily, depending on your size—but never more.

If you have over three drinks a day, your risk of developing liver disease and gastrointestinal cancer increases. Recent evidence links even moderate alcohol use to a 50 percent increase in breast cancer. Also, blood pressure starts to rise with anything over three drinks. In fact, excessive alcohol intake is one of the leading causes of elevated blood pressure.

If you drink alcohol for health purposes, it should be a prescription dose. Think of it like this: with prescription medicine, you would not skip your doses Monday to Thursday then take all those pills on Friday and Saturday to make up for it. It doesn't work that way. You cannot add up your doses and use them all on the same day. That is dangerous and the sign of a problem.

A Model of Moderation

That's enough with the disclaimers. For some people, alcohol can provide protective benefits. Although the degree of protection against cardiovascular disease varies from study to study, it is related to achieving the right dose. In the physicians' health study, light drinkers had a 28 percent decline in mortality (this was defined as only two to four drinks a week). Moderate drinker (five to six drinks a week) had a 21 percent decline in mortality. Heavy drinkers (more than six drinks weekly) actually had a 51 percent *increase* in mortality.

In other studies, alcohol was found to have stronger protective effects. One to three drinks daily lowered heart attack risk by about 50 percent. On the other hand, other causes of death increased with progressive intake.

Similar trends were noted in stroke prevention. Rare drinkers (one per month) had 62 percent fewer strokes. Those who had up to two drinks a day reduced stroke risk by 45 percent. And those who had five or more drinks daily *multiplied* their risk of stroke by three. So, as you can see, the dose is absolutely critical.

The correct amount of alcohol is actually pretty small. If you are having more than one or two drinks a day, check your motives. You are probably not doing it for your health.

The benefits also vary according to the type of alcoholic beverage you consume. Wine has the best results in optimal doses, with health risks reduced by 52 percent. Beer and spirits show a reduction of risk in the 45 percent range. However, in some studies, beer is shown as the least beneficial of alcoholic beverages.

There could be several reasons for this. One is the plant origin of the beverage. Wine is derived from colorful grapes that have heart protective flavonoids; beer and spirits are generally derived from less colorful grains that have fewer flavonoids.

Another possible explanation is the type of sugar involved. Grapes provide fruit sugar (fructose); the grains in beer and spirits provide maltose, which has a much higher glycemic index. In fact, it is one of the highest glycemic index foods out there. The result from consuming the maltose in beer is an insulin surge followed by fat accumulation. Is it any wonder that abdominal fat is called a beer belly?

Beer does tend to get stored as dangerous fat around the middle, predisposing a person to cardio-metabolic syndrome. As it turns out, heavy drinkers of any kind of alcohol have a higher risk of cardio-metabolic syndrome overall. Alcohol in high doses provides no health benefits—only excess calories that shut down weight loss and promote abdominal gain.

The body immediately turns off any fat burning process when alcohol enters the system. Its first priority is to rid the body of the toxin, so only after alcohol is removed can the fat burning resume. Furthermore, drinkers tend to become less inhibited and consume larger amounts of food with alcohol. So if you are serious about losing weight, alcohol is not a good addition to your diet. It is recommended more for those who want its nutritional benefits.

People who enjoy an occasional alcoholic beverage, particularly red wine, will see some cardiovascular effects from flavonoids. If you are someone who can accomplish this dietary addition safely and your main objective is not weight loss, then alcohol provides some health-preserving benefits to your daily program. However, if you do not have the right constitution for alcohol, then consider grape juice, apples, tea, chocolate, or other flavonoid sources and simply skip the booze.

Chapter 21: The Egg—Innocent or Guilty?

The poor egg has been pointed to with disdain for decades. People have scorned it for fear of damaging their hearts. Is this cholesterol-rich food really at fault, or is it simply guilty of hanging out with the wrong crowd, like its friends fried bacon, sausage, and buttered toast? Let us examine the facts to find out if we should really avoid eggs or if we're just being chicken.

The egg stands accused because of its high cholesterol content (about 213 mg each). But is high-cholesterol intake always bad? Most people certainly believe so—and it makes sense, doesn't it? If your arteries clog with cholesterol, then putting more in would aggravate the problem, right?

That's what the food industry wants us to believe. They have caught on to the public's cholesterol phobia and are more than willing to sell us food without it. In fact, "cholesterol-free" has become the new catch phrase.

The Shell Game

Shoppers grab food with a "no cholesterol" label; feeling assured that they are consuming something good for them. But are they being deceived? It is a little-known fact that cholesterol intake is *not* the strongest influence on blood cholesterol levels. It actually turns out that if cholesterol can be modified by diet, it is largely through the restriction of saturated fat and trans-fatty acids. These two components are the strongest elevators of cholesterol levels in the body. So a food labeled with "no cholesterol" could be full of saturated fats that actually *raise* cholesterol! Isn't that akin to false advertising?

Eggs, for one thing, are not the only source of cholesterol in the diet. Table 11 lists the cholesterol content in high-cholesterol foods (per milligram):

Table 11: Foods with High Cholesterol Content

Egg yolk: 213
Shrimp: 165
Beef, chicken, or pork: 70–85
Fish, lobster, clams (3 oz.): 50–60
Whole milk: 30–35
Cheese: 25–30
Non-fat milk: 10
Butter: 10
Egg white: 0

It's interesting that fish has moderate amounts of cholesterol, yet we have seen that eating fish regularly is associated with lower risk of heart disease. That seems somewhat contradictory, doesn't it? Here you are eating a food rich in cholesterol and at the same time lowering your risk of heart disease. This just goes to show that cholesterol is not all bad.

A similar study has been done with shrimp, which is somewhat infamous for its cholesterol content. However, a diet rich in shrimp did not show harmful results—but the *method* of preparation is important to consider. Fried shrimp, like anything else fried, has other dangers involved.

What do studies say about eggs? The short answer is, "That depends." For example, the Japanese have the lowest heart disease rate *and* the highest per capita egg consumption, averaging over six eggs a week per individual.

The Health Effects of Eggs
The majority of people (around 85 percent) are little affected by high cholesterol intake. For most patients, their blood

cholesterol will remain unchanged or go up minimally (around ten points) if cholesterol intake is increased. For those who are not overly responsive to the effects of cholesterol (which is the majority of the population), even massive amounts of it (more than 600 mg daily) produce no effects.

There are some exceptions, especially those who have inherited extremely high cholesterol levels. About 15 percent of these people are unable to excrete excess cholesterol because of their metabolism and can therefore see a significant increase in their blood cholesterol levels if they have high dietary cholesterol intakes.

So should we label all cholesterol intakes as bad for all people? I certainly think not. And should we continue to eschew the egg? No, because there are some positive things to be said for this food. It contains a very low amount of saturated fat (only about 1.6 grams), is high in protein, and low in carbohydrates. Eggs are also filling, which means they relieve hunger for prolonged periods of time while providing nutrition. That makes them an excellent food to promote weight reduction.

However, it is always a good idea to know and keep track of your cholesterol. If you are planning to make major dietary changes and perhaps utilize eggs as a tool in your diet, I recommend that you check your cholesterol both before and two to three months after beginning these changes to see how your body is responding. Many people (as much as 90 percent) will see a dramatic reduction in their cholesterol with the weight loss program I have outlined.

If you have a history of elevated cholesterol, you should exercise caution before adopting a long-term diet that is high in cholesterol. Instead, focus on favorable fats, like omega-3 and monosaturated fats, that are strong cholesterol reducers.

As always, a diet rich in natural, nutritious foods is your best option to maintain lean health—which means you can eat a few eggs without having to worry about walking on eggshells.

Chapter 22: Alternative Treatments

By now you realize that there is no substitute or shortcut for adopting lifestyle changes. Any health or weight loss intervention that does not include serious attempts to modify your lifestyle for the long term is doomed to failure.

But what are the options for the morbidly obese, who have more than a hundred pounds to lose, or those already suffering serious complications from their obesity, such as diabetes, heart conditions, or activity-limiting arthritis? Is there any hope for these extreme cases? Yes, there are a few options.

Help—and Hope—When You Need It

One of the miracle treatments for these advanced conditions is bariatric surgery to treat obesity. There are several varieties of this surgery, the mildest of which is gastric banding. Next comes vertical banded gastroplasty, and lastly, gastric bypass surgery. Without getting too technical (you obviously need to consult a doctor), I'd like to say that they are all extremely effective. Your weight can initially drop 20 to 30 percent and can be maintained within that range for the long run.

The metabolic effects of these treatments can also be fabulous. In addition to improving one's well-being and energy, these surgeries give patients better long-term odds of living (in the short term, there is a surgical risk of death of about 0.5 percent). Diabetes can be sent into remission, cardio-metabolic syndrome can be resolved completely, blood pressure drops significantly, and HDL cholesterol improves. Overall, bariatric surgery can be a life-altering procedure for those who are desperate. But these treatments do not preclude the aforementioned lifestyle changes. After surgery, a healthy diet and exercise should be adopted to ensure better chances of success.

Another option is metformin, a medicine that has recently been studied as a diabetic treatment. It has been shown to assist in weight loss, improve cardio-metabolic syndrome, and help prevent diabetes. Although it may cause side effects like nausea and diarrhea, it is worth considering if you are severely obese.

On the horizon are some promising additions. Although the research is preliminary, there is an excellent study with the still unreleased medicine Empatic. Patients taking this medicine were able to lose 5—8 percent of their body weight without altering their diet or exercise program in a six-month trial. Those that stayed on the medicine longer had even more dramatic weight loss of 10 percent of body weight or more. Adding diet and exercise improved the results.

By now, I think you know that the benefits of healthy nutrition extend far beyond weight loss, and that regardless of your treatment method, adopting healthy and delicious lifestyles is essential for a healthy body.

I would also caution patients from jumping on the bandwagon for any miracle cure that arrives. We have learned from the lessons of Phen-Phen that there are risks involved with any new medication. The most prudent approach to solving long-term weight problems is long-term lifestyle changes.

One more choice is cholesterol medication, which does not promote weight loss but will cause dramatic improvements in your blood cholesterol levels and risk of heart disease. For those who are fighting a daily battle with cholesterol by severely restricting saturated fats, cholesterol medication can free you from this constant battle, stop your carbohydrate binging, and allow you to focus more on weight loss.

Again, however, medical alternatives and lifestyle changes are not mutually exclusive. One may help save your life; the other will surely enhance it.

Chapter 23: Sample Diet

The human diet is so variable that is impossible to mandate any specific meal plan on a long-term basis. If you utilize the concepts in this book, then you will consistently make better meal choices. The following is a suggested guideline for developing a meal plan. A wide variety of fruits, nuts, and vegetables are selected to illustrate the flexibility of the plan. Each individual will develop their own favorites and preferences. After you have retried the spectrum of fruits and vegetables available, feel free to substitute your own favorites into the plan.

Typical serving sizes are as follows. Nut snacks are defined as one ounce or one-quarter cup. Egg dishes contain two eggs. Main courses are six ounces. Vegetable and salad portions are unlimited. Fruit portions are one large piece of fruit, or one handful or about four ounces if you are consuming berries, grapes, or other smaller fruit.

Sunday

Breakfast	Scrambled Eggs with Cheese
	Grapefruit, Green Tea
Snack	Plum
Lunch	Greek Salad
Snack	Walnuts
Dinner	Roasted Peppers
	Salmon Mango
	Green Salad with Garlic-Dijon Vinaigrette

Monday

Breakfast	Fruit Salad
	Green Tea
Snack	Walnuts
Lunch	Leftover Salmon Mango
Snack	Macadamia Nuts
Diner	Cucumber Salad
	Green Beans and Tomatoes
	Orange Chicken
Snack	Apple

Tuesday

Breakfast	Fruit Salad or Hard-Boiled Eggs
	Green Tea
Snack	Deluxe Mixed Nuts
Lunch	Rotisserie Chicken
	Sweet Potatoes, Salad
Snack	Orange
Diner	Wife's Killer Salad
	Seafood Stuffed Eggplant
Snack	Chocolate Covered Macadamia Nuts

Wednesday

Breakfast	Low Fat Yogurt with Fruit
	Green Tea, Banana, Grape Juice
Snack	Walnuts
Lunch	Leftovers or Replacement Meal
	Apple
Snack	Pear
Diner	Zucchini and Summer Squash
	Meatloaf (reduced calorie)
	Strawberries
Snack	Walnuts

Thursday

Breakfast	Low Fat Cottage Cheese
	Green Tea, Assorted Berries
Snack	Chocolate Cashews
Lunch	Spinach Salad
	Grapes
Snack	Walnuts
Diner	Garlic Spinach
	Herb Roasted Chicken
	Citrus Salad
Snack	Tangerine

Friday

Breakfast	Oat Bran
	Green Tea, Grape Juice
Snack	Deluxe Mixed Nuts
Lunch	Tuna Sandwich Whole Grain Bread
	Mustard, Tomatoes,
Snack	Plum
Diner	Grilled Sweet Potatoes
	Lentil Turkey Kielbasa Stew
	Cherries or Berries
Snack	Chocolate Almonds

Saturday

Breakfast	Cheese Omelet
	Green Tea, Melons, Orange Juice
Snack	Pistachios
Lunch	Tuna Salad or Leftovers
	Orange
Snack	Apple
Diner	Smothered Okra with Tomatoes
	Creole Scallops
Snack	Fruit Salad

Conclusion

The world is experiencing an epidemic of obesity, cardio-metabolic syndrome, diabetes, and other complications of weight gain. This spread of disease cannot be solved by short-term changes in behavior when faulty lifestyles are the foundation of the problem.

However, there is hope. It is possible to effectively change habits and develop better lifestyles—and this long-term change is a journey that will provide you with abundant health, energy, and happiness.

We've seen that one root of the problem is sedentary lifestyles. Overdependence on cars and passive amusements (such as TV and videogames) are eroding our health; we've got to stay active in order to survive! And that goes double for our younger generations.

The explosion of cheap, processed carbohydrate-concentrated foods is another social ill. Fast food restaurants should be named "fat food" restaurants to tell it like it is. It also hasn't helped that the public has been misinformed for decades about the supposed health benefits of the AHA recommended low-fat and high-carbohydrate diet, which has only aggravated the obesity problem.

Carbohydrate restriction is the most effective long-term weight loss program, but the popular Atkins philosophy has serious health flaws. Carbohydrates that are nutrient rich, as well as natural foods like fruits and vegetables, should not be restricted and replaced with saturated fats. Instead, medical professionals should be touting a diet steeped in healthier monosaturated fats and omega-3 sources, such as fish and nuts. (Most fad diets, however, are just plain fishy or nutty.)

How you prepare foods is almost as important as the food choices you make. Improper use of cooking oils, for instance, can thwart any attempts at healthy eating, particularly if trans-fatty acids are involved. And our country's obsession with frying should give way to flavonoids, food's hidden miracle and medicine's new frontier.

Redefining your identity is the key to affecting these essential lifestyle changes. You've got to start seeing yourself as an active, health-conscious individual and making choices that reaffirm that image. You also need to realize that exercising and eating healthily are not draconian punishments and that diet is not a "four-letter word." In fact, by following the Globe's Best Diet, you'll learn that eating well can be a rich and pleasurable experience that provides you with energy for living to your fullest.

Even when it comes to weight loss, there is so much to gain, like self-worth, new taste sensations, and a renewed sense of life—so start making changes today!

Recipes

Preparing a large fresh fruit salad (enough to last for two days) is easier than you might think. Think of the time saved for breakfast alone when you can just reach into the bowl and take out the ready prepared fruit of choice for each individual. Just be sure to keep it tightly covered to preserve freshness.

FRESH FRUIT SALAD

½ of a fresh small watermelon
½ of a cantaloupe
½ of a honeydew melon
1-pound strawberries
1 kiwi, sliced

Dice melons, carefully toss together, and add strawberries and kiwi on top.

Other fruits can be added or substituted as desired—blueberries, blackberries, pineapple, papaya, or any other type of melon of your choice. When melon quality looks a little undesirable a nice citrus salad can be made instead.

CITRUS SALAD

2 grapefruit, peeled and cut into segments
2–3 oranges, peeled and cut into segments
Kiwi, peeled and sliced for garnish
Any other seasonal fruit of choice
Banana, nuts

Prepare grapefruit and orange segments. Add other seasonal fruit of choice (grapes, berries, etc.). Toss to combine. Add banana only at serving time and sprinkle with nuts.

GREEK SALAD

3 medium tomatoes cut into wedges
1 medium cucumber, thinly sliced
1 small red onion, thinly sliced
2 tablespoons lemon juice
2 tablespoons olive oil
1 teaspoon snipped fresh oregano
Salt and pepper to taste
10 pitted kalamata olives
½ cup crumbled feta cheese

Combine the tomatoes, cucumber and red onion in a salad bowl. In a small bowl combine the lemon juice, olive oil, oregano and salt and pepper. Pour over the vegetables and toss lightly to combine. Allow to marinate until serving time. Top with olives and feta cheese.

Note: If you do not care for oregano, try Mrs. Dash "Garlic and Herbs" seasoning mix.

WIFE'S SALAD

4 cups of mixed greens
8 cherry tomatoes cut into halves
1 medium cucumber, thinly sliced
2 green onions, sliced
2 tablespoons balsamic vinegar
2 tablespoons olive oil
1 teaspoon snipped fresh cilantro
Salt and pepper to taste
½ cup crumbled gorgonzola cheese

Combine mixed greens, tomatoes, cucumber and green onion in a salad bowl. In a small bowl combine the vinegar, olive oil, salt and pepper. Pour over the vegetables and toss lightly to combine. Allow to marinate until serving time. Top with cilantro and gorgonzola cheese.

GREENS

When it comes to greens, you don't have to limit yourself to spinach and broccoli rabe. There are so many more, like kale, Swiss chard, escarole, mustard greens, turnip greens, and collards. Also, baby spinach makes a wonderful salad, as does arugula and romaine. And don't forget about broccoli and cauliflower.

ZUCCHINI AND YELLOW SUMMER SQUASH

These are both fast and easy to prepare. Choose small, firm squash. Wash thoroughly, thinly slice, and place in a microwave-safe container. Sprinkle with a little salt and pepper; add a small amount of olive oil, cover and microwave about 3 minutes, or until crisp-tender. Remove from microwave and sprinkle with Parmesan cheese. No need to add water when cooked in microwave as young squash has a high water content.

Legumes are a good source of protein and a good substitute for meat. Dried beans are not really difficult to prepare but slightly time consuming. For that purpose, the recipes below use canned beans—just make sure to rinse and drain to wash away excess sodium.

VEGETARIAN CHILI

1 medium onion, chopped
2 cloves garlic, minced
2 tablespoons canola oil
1 can (8 oz.) can tomato sauce
½ teaspoon dried oregano
2 cans (15 oz.) beans (kidney or pinto)
 rinsed and drained
Bottled hot pepper sauce, to taste (optional)

1 can (14½-oz.) stewed tomatoes
1 can beef broth (12oz.)
2 teaspoons chili powder
½ teaspoon cumin

In a large saucepan, heat oil and sauté onion until softened. Add garlic and continue to cook only about thirty seconds. Add remaining ingredients. Bring to boiling point; reduce heat to simmer and cook for about thirty minutes to blend flavors.

MINESTRONE (WITHOUT THE PASTA)

3 cans (14 oz.) beef broth (low sodium)
1 can (29 oz.) stewed tomatoes, undrained
1 can (6 oz.) tomato paste
1 can (15 oz.) red kidney beans, rinsed and drained
1 can (15 oz.) garbanzo beans, rinsed and drained
1 teaspoon dried Italian seasoning
2 cups frozen mixed vegetables (Italian blend)
1 cup fresh spinach leaves, cut into strips
Parmesan cheese, grated

In large saucepan, combine broth, tomatoes, sauce, beans and Italian seasoning. Bring to boiling; add frozen vegetables. Reduce heat to simmer, cover and cook until vegetables are tender. Add spinach just before serving. Serve with grated Parmesan, if desired.

This dish is better if made in advance to allow the flavors to blend. Reheat just before serving.

This recipe uses dry lentils, which requires less cooking time than most legumes. Leftovers can be frozen for another meal.

LENTIL, TURKEY KIELBASA STEW

1 medium onion, chopped
1 cup carrots, sliced
2 stalks celery, sliced
2 tablespoons canola oil
3 cloves garlic, minced
1 can (14 oz.) chicken broth
4 cups water
1 can (14 oz.) diced tomatoes
2 cups lentils (picked over and rinsed to remove any grit)
1-pound turkey kielbasa, cut into slices

In a large saucepot, heat the canola oil and add the onions, carrots and celery; cook until softened (about ten minutes) add garlic and cook another minute.

Add water, broth, tomatoes and lentils. Bring to boil, lower heat to a simmer, cover, and cook until lentils are tender (thirty-five—forty minutes). Add sliced turkey kielbasa during last ten minutes of cooking.

MANGOS—How to Prepare for Salsa

Cut mangos lengthwise in half, sliding sharp knife along flat side of the seed on each side, which will give you two large pieces. Cut away any remaining flesh from seed. Make crisscross pattern with knife on each half, then turn mango half inside out to cut off mango pieces.

MANGO SALSA

2 medium mangos, peeled and chopped
1 jalapeno, finely chopped
¼ cup lemon juice
¼ cup cilantro, chopped, or use flat leaf parsley

Remove ribs and seeds of jalapeno and chop finely. Combine all ingredients, cover and refrigerate until ready to use. Great on grilled, baked, or poached salmon.

MANGO-AVOCADO SALSA

1 medium mango, peeled and chopped   ¼ cup chopped red pepper
1 avocado, peeled and chopped   1 clove garlic, minced
2 teaspoons lime juice
½ of a jalapeno, seeded and finely chopped
¼ teaspoon salt
Combine ingredients, cover, and refrigerate until ready for use. Great with any type of fish.

MANGO-CUCUMBER SALSA

1½ cups diced mango
¾ cup diced cucumber (peeled and seeded)
½ cup diced red onion
1 jalapeno, finely diced
3 tablespoons lime juice
½ cup chopped flat leaf parsley
½ teaspoon salt
Mix ingredients and refrigerate to allow ingredients to blend.

MEAT LOAF (REDUCED CALORIE)

1 slice whole grain bread	1 egg (or 2 egg whites)
1 pound ground turkey	½ small onion, chopped
½ pound ground beef or ground pork	1 clove garlic, minced
¼ cup ketchup	2 teaspoons Worchestershire sauce

Toss slice of bread into blender or food processor to make crumbs.
Combine ingredients and form into loaf. Bake at 350° for thirty–
forty minutes. Instant-read thermometer should register 160°.

APRICOT-DIJON CHICKEN (no added fat)

4 boneless, skinless chicken breasts
(if desired use bone-in chicken thighs, but remove skin)
Salt & pepper to taste   ½ cup apricot preserves
1 tablespoon Dijon mustard
½ teaspoon ground ginger
½ teaspoon garlic powder
2 tablespoons ketchup

Sprinkle chicken with salt and pepper and place in large plastic
bag. Combine remaining ingredients and pour over chicken.
Marinate for at least 2 hours. Heat oven to 375°. Place chicken in

baking dish. Bake approximately twenty-five minutes for breasts, thirty–thirty-five for thighs. If desired, toasted chopped walnuts could be sprinkled over top.

ORANGE CHICKEN

6 bone-in chicken thighs, skin removed
2 navel oranges (1 for juice and grated rind, the other for slicing)
1 teaspoon honey
½ teaspoon ground ginger

Combine juice from one orange, the grated orange rind, honey, and ginger. Place chicken in roasting pan, pour mixture over, and allow to marinate for about twenty minutes. Thinly slice remaining orange and arrange over chicken. Cook in oven for about thirty minutes at 350°.

HERB-ROASTED CHICKEN

1 3 to 3½-pound whole broiler chicken
1 tablespoon olive oil
2 cloves garlic, minced
¼ teaspoon salt
¼ teaspoon lemon-pepper seasoning
½ teaspoon each ground sage and dried thyme

Rinse inside of chicken and pat dry. Brush chicken with olive oil; rub garlic over chicken. Combine dry spices; sprinkle some inside chicken cavity, and brush remainder over chicken. Roast, uncovered, in a 350° for about one to one-and-a-half hours (180° on meat thermometer). Remove from oven, cover chicken, and allow to rest for ten minutes before carving.

For the freshest and best quality of most vegetables, a visit to a local farmers market could be a delightful surprise along with very reasonable prices.

ROASTED RED PEPPERS

Ingredients are nothing but peppers.

The simplest method to prepare is to cut the raw peppers in half, remove seeds, and place them, cut side down, on a sheet pan (line sheet pan with foil for easy clean-up). Broil until blackened, remove from oven, and place them in a large bowl. Cover bowl and allow them to rest until cool enough to handle. Blackened skin will then slide right off. You will be surprised at the amount of oil from the peppers that accumulates in the bowl.

It is as simple as that! Can be used as a side dish or an appetizer or as an ingredient in pasta sauce—or just be creative.

ROASTED RED PEPPER DIP

4 red peppers, roasted (as above)
½ cup whole almonds
1 teaspoon red wine vinegar
3 tablespoons olive oil

2 garlic cloves
1 teaspoon salt
¼ teaspoon paprika

Spread almonds on baking sheet and bake at 350° until golden, cool. In food processor, puree roasted red peppers, nuts garlic, salt, vinegar, and paprika. Add oil and process until smooth. Garnish with fresh chopped parsley. If desired, a touch of fresh chopped mint leaves can be added.

ROAST TOMATO APPETIZER

8 plum tomatoes
Olive oil
1 can artichoke bottoms
16 small mozzarella balls
Pesto

Cut tomatoes in half, remove seeds and juice. Brush with olive oil. Roast in slow oven (250°) approximately one hour. Drain artichoke bottoms and place on baking sheet (cut off small portion of bottom so it can stand). Place half of roasted tomato on top of artichoke; add a small mozzarella ball and a bit of pesto on top. Bake in oven at 350° just long enough to warm thoroughly.

VEGETABLE SALAD WITH BROWN RICE

If time is an issue, instant brown rice can be used—or, leftover brown rice could be used. If desired, other vegetables can be substituted or added (celery, scallions, radishes).

1 cup cooked brown rice
1 plum tomato, diced
1 cucumber, peeled and diced
½ cup diced red onion
1 small head of romaine
Vinaigrette dressing

Make sure rice is cool before proceeding with salad. Line salad plate with romaine. Combine ingredients and add vinaigrette dressing, salt, and pepper to taste. Place on romaine lined salad plate.

SIMPLE VINAIGRETTE DRESSING

1 tablespoon red wine vinegar
3 tablespoons olive oil

Slowly whisk olive oil into vinegar.

Your own vinaigrette is easy to prepare without the added sugar and preservatives found in most bottled dressings. Dressings made with olive oil will thicken when chilled, when using it after the first day, allow it to stand at room temperature for about thirty minutes. Or, prepare a smaller quantity.

GARLIC-DIJON VINAIGRETTE

1 clove garlic, minced
4 tablespoons lemon juice
2 tablespoons Dijon mustard
2 tablespoons rice vinegar
Salt and pepper to taste
1-cup olive oil

Whisk all ingredients except oil in a small bowl (or use a blender). Slowly whisk in oil until thick vinaigrette is formed.

BALSAMIC VINAIGRETTE

1 clove garlic, minced
$1/_3$-cup balsamic vinegar
1 teaspoon Dijon mustard
Salt and pepper to taste
$1/_3$-cup olive oil

Combine first four ingredients, slowly whisk in olive oil. Any fresh or dried herb of your choice can be added.

SHRIMP CREOLE

1 large onion, chopped
1 green pepper, chopped
2 cloves garlic, minced
2 tablespoons canola oil
1 pound okra, sliced, <u>or</u> sliced frozen okra
1 can (28 oz.) chopped tomatoes with juice
2 pounds shelled shrimp
½ pound sliced mushrooms
1 tablespoon Creole seasoning
Hot paprika, salt and pepper to taste

Sauté onion and green pepper in canola oil until soft. Add garlic and continue to cook for another minute. Add tomatoes, okra, and seasoning; simmer until okra is tender. Just before serving, add shrimp and mushrooms; cook just until shrimp are done.

CREOLE SCALLOPS

1½ pounds sea scallops
2 tablespoons canola oil
2 tablespoons Creole seasoning
1 green pepper, chopped
1 large onion, chopped
2 stalks celery, chopped
2 cloves garlic, minced
1 can (14 oz.) chopped tomatoes
1-tablespoon tomato paste
Parsley

Season the scallops with 1 tablespoon of the Creole seasoning. Heat 1 tablespoon of the oil in large skillet and sauté the scallops for about 3 minutes per side; remove and reserve.

Add additional oil to skillet and sauté onion, pepper and celery until softened. Add garlic and cook for another minute. Add tomatoes, tomato paste and remaining Creole seasoning. Cover, and simmer for about 5 minutes. Return scallops to skillet and heat. Garnish with parsley.

GRILLED SWEET POTATOES

2 large sweet potatoes
2 tablespoons olive oil
Salt and pepper to taste
Peel sweet potatoes and cut into long wedges. Mix oil, salt, and pepper in a large bowl or plastic bag. Add potatoes and mix to coat. Cook on outside grill or stovetop grill (turning occasionally) until tender—approximately thirty minutes.

Note: Can also be baked in 400° oven on a foil-lined baking sheet (decrease olive oil to 1 tablespoon) for twenty-five to thirty minutes.

ESCAROLE AND MEATBALL SOUP

1 pound ground turkey
1 slice whole grain bread (made into breadcrumbs)
½ teaspoon Italian seasoning
2 tablespoons grated Parmesan cheese
Salt and pepper to taste
1-tablespoon canola oil
1 large onion, chopped
2 shredded carrots
2 cloves garlic, minced
4 cups chicken broth
1 bunch escarole, cleaned and cut into strips

Mix ground turkey, breadcrumbs, Italian seasoning, salt, pepper, and Parmesan cheese. Form into small meatballs and set aside. In a large saucepan, heat oil; add onion and carrots and sauté until onions are tender. Add garlic and sauté another minute; add chicken broth, escarole and meatballs. Simmer, covered for ten to fifteen minutes. Remove from heat and stir in additional Parmesan cheese.

TOMATO SALSA

3 medium tomatoes, seeded and finely chopped
$^1/_3$ cup finely chopped red onion
1 jalapeno pepper, seeded and finely chopped
2 tablespoons lime juice
2 cloves garlic
¼ teaspoon salt
1 tablespoon chopped cilantro or parsley
Combine all ingredients. Cover and chill for at least two hours.

CUCUMBER DILL SAUCE

1 medium cucumber, peeled and diced
1 cup plain low-fat yogurt
3 tablespoons chopped fresh dill
1 clove garlic, minced
Salt to taste

Combine ingredients; refrigerate at least thirty minutes for flavors to blend.

ROASTED ASPARAGUS

2 pounds asparagus
1½ tablespoons olive oil
Salt and pepper

Heat oven to 400°. Trim ends of asparagus. Place in single layer on a baking sheet. Drizzle with the olive oil and sprinkle with salt and pepper. Turn to coat and bake approximately eighteen minutes. If desired, strips of red and yellow peppers could be roasted along with asparagus.

GREEN BEANS

Green beans are great just steamed, with a little salt and pepper (if desired). Serve with a generous helping of sliced almonds on top and perhaps a squirt of lemon juice.

GREEN BEANS AND TOMATOES

1 pound fresh green beans, trimmed
1 pint grape tomatoes, halved
1 tablespoon lemon juice
2 tablespoons wine vinegar
¼ cup olive oil
Salt and pepper to taste
½ cup chopped walnuts

Cook beans in a small amount of salted water about ten to fifteen minutes or until tender. Drain and rinse under cool water, pat dry. Add grape tomatoes. Meanwhile prepare vinaigrette with vinegar, lemon juice, and olive oil; add to green bean mixture and toss to combine (best if allowed to marinate at least ½ hour). Top with chopped walnuts at serving time.

SMOTHERED OKRA AND TOMATOES

2 tablespoons canola oil
1 medium onion, chopped
1 green pepper, chopped
1 clove garlic, minced
2 cups fresh okra, sliced (or frozen)
2 cups fresh tomatoes, peeled and chopped,
 (Or 1 can (14 oz.) chopped tomatoes)
Salt and pepper to taste

In a large saucepan, sauté the onion and green pepper in the canola oil until tender. Add the garlic and continue to cook for another minute. Add remaining ingredients, bring to boil; reduce heat to a simmer. Cover and simmer until okra is tender, about twenty minutes.

Note: Good fresh okra is sometimes difficult to find; if they look shriveled, dark, or soft, choose frozen instead. Cooking time will possibly be shortened.

Bibliography

Adamcik, Raymond D. "A Case Report: Miracle HDL Diet." Unpublished case report, 2000.

Adams, Kenneth F., Arthur Schatzkin, Tamara B. Harris, Victor Kipnis, Traci Mouw, Rachel Ballard-Barbash, Albert Hollenbeck, and Michael F. Leitzmann. "Overweight, Obesity, and Mortality in a Large Prospective Cohort of Persons 50 to 71 Years Old." *New England Journal of Medicine* 355, no. 8 (2006): 763–78.

Adams, Stacy. "Inappropriate Drug Dosage in Obese Patients Cause for Alarm." *Endocrine Today*, January 2008, 40.

Almario, Rogelio, Veraphon Vonghavaravat, Rodney Wong, and Sidika E. Kasim-Karakas. "Effects of Walnut Consumption on Plasma Fatty Acids and Lipoproteins in Combined Hyperlipidemia." *American Journal of Clinical Nutrition 74*, no. 1 (July 2001): 72–9.

Alper, Phillip. "Is Internal Medicine in a Cyclical Downturn?" *Internal Medicine World Report*, December 2007.

Ambrose, Marietta, Christian Nagy, and Roger S. Blumenthal. "Relationships Exist Between Exercise Capacity, Physical Fitness, Adiposity and CVD Risk." *Endocrine Today*, February 25, 2008.

Anderson, Christopher B., Brian T. Helfand, and Kevin T. McVary. "Clinical Markers of Benign Prostaic Hyperplasia

Progression." *Weill Medical College of Cornell University Reports on Men's Urologic Health* 3, no. 1 (2008): 1–7.

Anderson, James W. "Office Management of the Overweight and Obese." *Primary Care Quarterly*, December 2007.

Appel, Lawrence J., Frank M. Sacks, Vincent J. Carey, Eva Obarzanek, Janis F. Swain, Edgar R. Miller, Paul R. Conlin, et al. "Effects of Protein, Monounsaturated Fat, and Carbohydrate Intake on Blood Pressure and Serum Lipids: Results of the OmniHeart Randomized Trial." *JAMA* 294, no. 19 (2005): 2455–64.

Arone, Louis J. "Cardiometabolic Risk: Finding a New Treatment Approach." *Baylor College of Medicine Reports on Cardiometabolic Disorders* 1, no. 4 (2007): 1–7.

Artaud-Wild, Sabine, Sonja L. Connor, Gary Sexton, William E. Connor. "Differences in Coronary Mortality Can Be Explained by Differences in Cholesterol and Saturated Fat Intakes in 40 Countries but Not in France and Finland: A Paradox." *Circulation* 88, no. 6 (December 1993): 2771–79.

Arts, Ilja C.W., Peter C.H. Hollman, Edith J.M. Feskens, H. Bas Bueno de Mesquita, and Daan Kromhout. "Catechin Intake Might Explain the Inverse Relation Between Tea Consumption and Ischemic Heart Disease: The Zutphen Elderly Study." *American Journal of Clinical Nutrition* 74, no. 2 (August 2001): 227–32.

Ascherio, Alberto, Charles H. Hennekens, Julie E. Buring, Carol Master, Meir J. Stampfer, and Walter C. Willett. "Trans-Fatty Acids Intake and Risk of Myocardial Infarction." *Circulation* 89, no. 1 (January 1994): 94–101.

Asghar, Rana Jawad, Robert H. Pratt, Steve Kammerer, and Thomas R. Navin. "Tuberculosis in South Asians Living in the United States, 1993–2004." *Archives of Internal Medicine* 168, no. 9 (May 12, 2008): 936–43.

Baker, Herman. "Nutrition in the Elderly: An Overview." *Geriatrics* 62, no. 7 (2007): 28–31.

Baker, Jennifer L., Lina W. Olsen, and Thorkild I. A. Sørensen. "Childhood Body-Mass Index and the Risk of Coronary Heart Disease in Adulthood." *New England Journal of Medicine* 357, no. 23 (2007): 2329–37.

Bates, Betsy. "Combat 'Diabesity' with Nutrition and Exercise." *Internal Medicine News* 41, no. 5 (2008): 28.

Baumel, Syd. "Deadly Donuts, Fatal Fries: Experts Blow Whistle on Diet's Direst Fat." The Aquarian. http://www.aquarianonline.com/Wellness/TransFatty.html (accessed 08/13/2002).

Bemelmans, Wanda J.E., Jan Broer, Edith J.M. Feskens, Andries J. Smit, Frits A.J. Muskiet, Johan D. Lefrandt, Victor J.J. Bom, Johan F. May, and Betty Meyboom-de Jong. "Effect of an Increased Intake of a-Linolenic Acid and Group Nutritional Education on Cardiovascular Risk Factors: The Mediterranean Alpha-Linolenic Enriched Groningen Dietary Intervention (MARGARIN) Study." *American Journal of Clinical Nutrition* 75, no. 2 (February 2002): 221–7.

Beulens, Joline W.J., and Yvonne T. van der Schouw. "Increased Risk of Cardiovascular Disease among Middle-Aged Women Due To Glycemic Load." *Cardiology Review*, February 2008.

Blackburn, George L., Judy C. C. Phillips, Susan Morreale. "Physician's Guide to Popular Low-Carbohydrate Weight-Loss Diets." *Cleveland Clinic Journal of Medicine* 68, no. 9 (September 2001): 761–74.

Bleys, Joachim, Ana Navas-Acien, and Eliseo Guallar. "Serum Selenium Levels and All-Cause, Cancer, and Cardiovascular Mortality Among US Adults." *Archives of Internal Medicine* 168, no. 4 (February 25, 2008): 404–10.

Bonanome, Andrea, and Scott M. Grundy. "Effect of Dietary Stearic Acid on Plasma Cholesterol and Lipoprotein Levels." *New England Journal of Medicine* 318, no. 19 (May 12, 1988): 1244–8.

Boschert, Sherry. "Diabetes Guidelines Contain Hidden Pearls of Nutritional Advice." *Internal Medicine News* 41, no. 6 (March 15, 2008): 13.

Boschert, Sherry. "Successful Weight Losers Use Similar Strategies." *Internal Medicine News* 41, no. 10 (May 15, 2008): 26.

Bravata, Dena M., Lisa Sanders, Jane Huang, Harlan M. Krumholz, Ingram Olkin, Christopher D. Gardner, and Dawn M. Bravata. "Efficacy and Safety of Low-Carbohydrate Diets: A Systematic Review." *JAMA* 289, no. 14 (April 9, 2003): 1837–50.

Brunk, Doug. "DASH Diet Shown to Lower Risk of Heart Disease and Stroke." *Internal Medicine News*, January 1, 2008, 35.

Burbank, Kelton M., J. Herbert Stevenson, Gregory R. Czarnecki, and Justin Dorfman. "Chronic Shoulder Pain: Part I. Evaluation and Diagnosis." *American Family Physician* 77, no. 4 (February 15, 2008): 453–60.

Burke, Gregory L., Alain G. Bertoni, Steven Shea, Russell Tracy, Karol E. Watson, Roger S. Blumenthal, Hyoju Chung, and Mercedes R. Carnethon. "The Impact of Obesity on Cardiovascular Disease Risk Factors and Subclinical

Vascular Disease." *Archives of Internal Medicine* 168, no. 9 (May 12, 2008): 928–34.

Burr, M.L., A.M. Fehily, J.F. Gilbert, S. Rogers, R.M. Holliday, P.M. Sweetnam, P.C. Elwood, N.M. Deadman. "Effects of Changes in Fat, Fish, and Fibre Intakes on Death and Myocardial Reinfarction: Diet and Reinfarction Trial (DART)." *The Lancet*, September 30, 1989 (8666): 757–61.

Chandalia, Manisha, Abhimanyu Garg, Dieter Lutjohann, Klaus von Bergmann, Scott M. Grundy, and Linda J. Brinkley. "Beneficial Effects of High Dietary Fiber Intake in Patients with Type 2 Diabetes Mellitus." *New England Journal of Medicine* 342, no. 19 (May 11, 2000): 1392–8.

Choi, Hyon K., Karen Atkinson, Elizabeth W. Karlson, Walter Willett, and Gary Curhan. "Purine-Rich Foods, Dairy and Protein Intake, and the Risk of Gout in Men." *New England Journal of Medicine* 350, no. 11 (2004): 1093–1103.

Cohn, Peter F. "Increased Glycemic Load: No Friend to Middle-Aged Women?" *Cardiology Review*, February 2008.

Cortlandt Forum. Quick Digest. December, 2007.

Curtis, Brian M., and James O'Keefe, Jr. "Understanding the Mediterranean Diet: Could This Be the New 'Gold Standard' for Heart Disease Prevention?" *Postgraduate Medicine* 112, no. 2 (August 2002): 35–45.

Dai, Qi, Amy Borenstein, Yougui Wu, James C. Jackson, and Eric B. Larson. "Fruit and Vegetable Juices and Alzheimer's Disease: The *Kame* Project." *American Journal of Medicine* 119 (2006): 751–59.

de Lorgeril, Michel, Patricia Salen, Jean-Louis Martin, Isabelle Monjaud, Jacques Delaye, and Nicole Mamelle. "Mediterranean Diet, Traditional Risk Factors, and the

Rate of Cardiovascular Complications after Myocardial Infarction." *Circulation* 99 (February 16, 1999): 779–85.

de Lorgeril, Michel, Patricia Salen, Jean-Louis Martin, Isabelle Monjaud, Philippe Boucher, and Nicole Mamelle. "Mediterranean Dietary Pattern in a Randomized Trial: Prolonged Survival and Possible Reduced Cancer Rate." *Archives of Internal Medicine* 158, no. 11 (June 8, 1998): 1181–7.

Denke, Margo A. "Diet, Lifestyle, and Nonstatin Trials: Review of Time to Benefit." *American Journal of Cardiology* 96, no. 5A (2005): 3F–10F.

Douglas, Mark. *Trading in the Zone: Master the Market with Confidence, Discipline and a Winning Attitude.* New York: New York Institute of Finance, 2000.

Dreon, Darlene M., Harriet A. Fernstrom, Hannia Campos, Patricia Blanche, Paul T. Williams, and Ronald M. Krauss. "Change in Dietary Saturated Fat Intake is Correlated with Change in Mass of Large Low-Density-Lipoprotein Particles in Men." *American Journal of Clinical Nutrition* 67, no. 4 (October 1998): 828–36.

Ebbesson, Sven O. E., M. Elzabeth Tejero, Elizabeth D. Nobmann, Juan Carlos Lopez-Alvarenga, Lars Ebbesson, Terri Romenesko, Elizabeth A. Carter, et al. "Fatty Acid Consumption and Metabolic Syndrome Components: The GOCADAN Study." *JCMS*, Fall 2007, 244–8.

Eckel, Robert H. "Nonsurgical Management of Obesity in Adults." *New England Journal of Medicine* 358, no. 18 (2008): 1941–50.

Elam, Marshall B., Donald B. Hunninghake, Kathryn B. Davis, Rekha Garg, Craig Johnson, Debra Egan, John B. Kostis, David S. Sheps, and Eliot A. Brinton. "Effect of Niacin on Lipid and Lipoprotein Levels and Glycemic Control in Patients with Diabetes and Peripheral Arterial Disease." *JAMA* 284, no. 10 (September 13, 2000): 1263–70.

Esposito, Katherine, Raffaele Marfella, Miryam Ciotola, Carmen Di Palo, Francesco Giugliano, Giovanni Giugliano, Massimo D'Armiento, Francesco D'Andrea, and Dario Giugliano. "Effect of a Mediterranean-Style Diet on Endothelial Dysfunction and Markers of Vascular Inflammation in the Metabolic Syndrome: A Randomized Trial." *JAMA* 292, no. 12 (2004): 1440–6.

Fletcher, Gerald, and Jorge F. Trejo. "Why and How to Prescribe Exercise: Overcoming the Barriers." *Cleveland Clinic Journal of Medicine* 72, no. 8 (August 2005): 645–56.

Folsom, Aaron R., Jing Ma, Paul C.McGovern, and John H. Eckfeldt. "Relation between Plasma Phospholipid Saturated Fatty Acids and Hyperinsulinemia." *Metabolism* 45, no. 2 (February 1996): 223–8.

Fonseca, Vivian A. "Identification and Treatment of Prediabetes to Prevent Progression of Type 2 Diabetes." *Clinical Cornerstone* 8, no. 2 (2007): 10–20.

Foreyt, John P. "Need for Lifestyle Intervention: How to Begin." *American Journal of Cardiology* 96, supplement (2005): 11E–14E.

Foster, Gary D., Holly R. Wyatt, James O. Hill, Brian G. McGuckin, Carrie Brill, Selma Mohammed, Philippe O. Szapary, Daniel J. Rader, Joel S. Edman, and Samuel Klein. "A Randomized Trial of a Low-Carbohydrate Diet for Obesity." *New England Journal of Medicine* 348, no. 21 (May 22, 2003): 2082–90.

Foster-Powell, Kaye, Susanna H.A. Holt, and Janette Brand-Miller. "International Table of Glycemic Index and

Glycemic Load Values: 2002." *American Journal of Clinical Nutrition* 76, no. 1 (July 2002): 5–56.

Fung, Teresa, Stephanie E. Chiuve, Marjorie L. McCullough, Kathryn M. Rexrode, Giancarlo Logroscino, and Frank B. Hu. "Adherence to a DASH_Style Diet and Risk of Coronary Heart Disease and Stroke in Women." *Archives of Internal Medicine* 168, no. 7 (April 14, 2008): 713–20.

Galor, A., and B.H. Jeng. "Red Eye for the Internist: When to Treat, When to Refer." *Cleveland Clinic Journal of Medicine* 75, no. 2 (February 2008): 137–44.

Gardner, Christopher D., Alexandre Kiazand, Sofiya Alhassan, Soowon Kim, Randall S. Stanford, Raymond R. Balise, Helena C. Kraemer, and Abby C. King. "Comparison of the Atkins, Zone, Ornish, and LEARN Diets for Change in Weight and Related Risk Factors among Overweight Premenopausal Women. The A to Z Wight Loss Study: An Randomized Trial." *JAMA* 297, no. 9 (2007): 969–77.

Gaziano, J.M., C.H. Hennekens, S.L. Godfried, H.D. Sesso, R.J. Glynn, J.L. Breslow, and J.E. Buring. "Type of Alcoholic Beverage and Risk of Myocardial Infarction." *American Journal of Cardiology* 83, no. 1 (January 1999): 52–7.

Glueck, Charles J. "Dietary Fat and Atherosclerosis." *American Journal of Clinical Nutrition* 32, no. 12 (December 1979): 2703–11.

Gregg, Edward W., Jane A. Cauley, Katie Stone, Theodore J. Thompson, Douglas C. Bauer, Steven R. Cummings, and Kristine E. Ensrud. "Relationship of Changes in Physical Activity and Mortality Among Older Women." *JAMA* 289, no. 18 (May 14, 2003): 2379–86.

Gregg, Edward W., Robert B. Gerzoff, Carl J. Caspersen, David F. Williamson, and K. M. Venkat Narayan. "Relationship of Walking to Mortality Among U.S. Adults with Diabetes." *Archives of Internal Medicine* 163, no. 12 (June 23, 2003): 1440–7.

Grundy, Scott. "The Optimal Ratio of Fat-to-Carbohydrate in the Diet." *Annual Review of Nutrition* 19 (1999): 325–41.

Grundy, Scott, Henry Y. I. Mok, Loren Zech, and Mones Berman. "Influence of Nicotine Acid on Metabolism of Cholesterol and Triglycerides in Man." *Journal of Lipid Research* 22, no. 1 (January 1981): 24–36.

Haffner, Steven M., Rodolfo A. Valdez, Helen P. Hazuda, Braxton D. Mitchell, Phillip A. Morales, and Michael P. Stern. "Prospective Analysis of the Insulin-Resistance Syndrome (SyndromeX)." *Diabetes* 41, no.6 (June 1992): 715–21.

Halton, Thomas L., Walter C. Willett, Simin Liu, JoAnn E. Manson, Christine M. Albert, Kathryn Rexrode, and Frank B. Hu. "Low-Carbohydrate-Diet Score and the Risk of Coronary Heart Disease in Women." *New England Journal of Medicine* 355, no. 19 (2006): 1991–2002.

Harper, Charles R., and Terry A. Jacobson. "Usefulness of Omega-3 Fatty Acids and the prevention of Coronary Heart Disease." *American Journal of Cardiology* 96, no. 11 (2005): 1521–9.

Harper, Charles R., and Terry A. Jacobson. "The Fats of Life: The Role of Omega-3 Fatty Acids in the Prevention of Coronary Heart Disease." *Archives of Internal Medicine* 161, no. 18 (October 8, 2001): 2185–92.

Harris, William S. "Fish Oil Supplementation: Evidence for Health Benefits." *Cleveland Clinic Journal of Medicine* 71, no. 3 (2004): 208–20.

He, Ka, Eric B. Rimm, Anwar Merchant, Bernard A. Rosner, Meir J. Stampfer, Walter C. Willett, and Alberto Ascherio. "Fish Consumption and Risk of Stroke in Men." *JAMA* 288, no. 24 (December 25, 2002): 3130–6.

HealthCheck Systems. "Understanding Fat and Cholesterol." HealthCheck Systems. http://www.healthchecksystems. com/chol.htm (accessed 07/04/2000).

Hertog, Michael G. L., Daan Kromhout, Christ Aravanis, Henry Blackburn, Ratko Buzina, Flaminio Fidanza, Simona Giampaoli, Annemarie Jansen, Alessandro Menotti, Srecko Nedeljkovic, Marija Pekkarinen, Bozidar S. Simic, Hironori Toshima, Edith J. M. Feskins, Peter C. H. Hollman, Martijn B. Katan. "Flavinoid Intake and Long-Term Risk of Coronary Heart Disease and Cancer in the Seven Countries Study." *Archives of Internal Medicine* 155, no. 4 (February 27, 1995): 381–6.

Heyden, Siegfried. "Polyunsaturated and Monounsaturated Fatty Acids in the Diet to Prevent Coronary Heart Disease via Cholesterol Reduction." *Annals of Nutrition and Metabolism* 38, no. 3 (1994): 117–22.

Higdon, Jane. "Micronutrient Information Center: Glycemic Index and Glycemic Load. Linus Pauling Institute at Oregon State University. http://lpi.oregonstate.edu/ infocenter/foods/grains/gigl.html(accessed 04/17/2008).

Horvath, Karl, Klaus Jeitler, Ulrich Siering, Anne K. Stich, Guido Skipka, Thomas W. Gratzer, and Andrea Siebenhofer. "Long-Term Effects of Weight-Reducing Interventions in

Hypertensive Patients." *Archives of Internal Medicine* 168, no. 6 (March 24, 2008): 571–80.

Hu, Frank B. "The Mediterranean Diet and Mortality – Olive Oil and Beyond." *New England Journal of Medicine* 348, no. 26 (June 26, 2003): 2595–6.

Hu, Frank B., Leslie Bronner, Walter C. Willett, Meir J. Stampfer, Kathryn M. Rexrode, Christine M. Albert, David Hunter, and JoAnn E. Manson. "Fish and Omega-3 Fatty Acid Intake and Risk of Coronary Heart Disease in Women." *JAMA* 287, no. 14 (April 10, 2002): 1815–21.

Hu, Frank B., JoAnn E. Manson, Meir J. Stampfer, Graham Colditz, Simin Liu, Caren G. Solomon, and Walter C. Willett. "Diet, Lifestyle, and the Risk of Type 2 Diabetes Mellitus in Women." *New England Journal of Medicine* 345, no. 11 (September 13, 2001): 790–7.

Hu, Frank B., Meir J. Stampfer, Graham A. Colditz, Alberto Ascherio, Kathryn M. Rexrode, Walter C. Willett, JoAnn E. Manson. "Physical Activity and Risk of Stroke in Women." *JAMA* 283, no. 2 (June 14, 2000): 2961–7.

Iso, Hiroyasu, Kathryn M. Rexode, Meir J. Stampfer, JoAnn E. Manson, Graham A. Colditz, Frank E. Speizer, Charles H. Hennekens, and Walter C. Willett. "Intake of Fish and Omega-3 Fatty Acids and Risk of Stroke in Women." *JAMA* 285, no. 3 (January 17, 2001): 304–12.

Jackson, Rod, Joanna Broad, Jennie Connor, and Susan Wells. "Alcohol and Ischaemic Heart Disease: Probably No Free Lunch." *Lancet* 366 (December 2005): 1911–2.

Jenkins, D.J., D.G. Popovich, C.W. Kendall, E. Vidgen, N. Tariq, T.P. Ransom, T.M. Wolever, V. Vuksan, C.C. Melding, D.L. Boctor, C. Bolognesi, J. Huang, and R. Patten. "Effect of a Diet High in Vegetables, Fruit, and

Nuts on Serum Lipids." *Metabolism* 46, no. 5 (May 1997): 530–7.

Jiang, Rui, JoAnn E. Manson, Meir J. Stampfer, Simin Liu, Walter C. Willett, Frank B. Hu. "Nut and Peanut Butter Consumption and Risk of Type 2 Diabetes in Women." *JAMA* 288, no. 20 (2002): 2554–60.

Kalvaitis, Katie. "Western Diet Increased Risk for Developing Metabolic Syndrome." *Endocrine Today*, March 25, 2008.

Katan, Martijn B., Peter L. Zock and Ronald B. Mensink. "Trans Fatty Acids and Their Effects on Lipoproteins in Humans." *Annual Review of Nutrition* 15 (1995): 474–91.

Keenan, J.M., J.B. Wenz, S. Myers, C. Ripsin, and Z.Q. Huang. "Randomized, Controlled, Crossover Trial of Oat Bran in Hypercholesterolemic Subjects." *Journal of Family Practice* 33, no. 6 (December 1991): 600–8.

Keller, Daniel M. "The HDL-C Conundrum: When More of the 'Good' Isn't So Great." *Internal Medicine World Report*, July 2007.

Kestin, Mark, Peter Clifton, G. Bryan Belling, and Paul J. Nestel. "n-3 Fatty Acids of Marine Origin Lower Systolic Blood Pressure and Triglycerides but Raise LDL Cholesterol Compared with n-3 and n-6 Fatty Acids From Plants." *American Journal of Clinical Nutrition* 51, no. 6 (June 1990): 1028–34.

Keys, Ancel, Alessandro Menotti, Martti Karvonen, Christ Aravanis, Henry Blackburn, Ratko Buzina, R.S. Djordjevic, A.S. Dontas, Flaminio Fidanza, Margaret Keys, Daan Kromhout, Srecko Nedeljkovic, Sven Punsar, Fulvia Seccareccia, and Hironori Toshima. "The Diet and 15-Year Death Rate in the Seven Countries Study." *American Journal of Epidemiology* 124, no. 6 (1986): 903–13.

Kim, Alice, and Thomas Keys. "Infective Endocarditis Prophylaxis before Dental Procedures: New Guidelines Spark Controversy." *Cleveland Clinic Journal of Medicine* 75, no. 2 (2008): 89–92.

Knoops, Kim T. B., Lisette C. P. G. G. M. de Groot, Daan Kromhout, Anne-Elisabeth Perrin, Olga Moreiras-Varela, Alessandro Menotti, and Wija A. van Staveren. "Mediterranean Diet, Lifestyle Factors, and 10-Year Mortality in Elderly European Men and Women: The HALE Project." *JAMA* 292, no. 12 (2004): 1433–8.

Kontogianni, Meropi D., Demosthenes B. Panagiotakos, Christina Chrysohoou, Christos Pitsavos, Antonis Zampelas, and Christodoulos Stefanadis. "The Impact of Olive Oil Consumption Pattern on the Risk of Acute Coronary Syndromes: The Cardio2000 Case—Control Study." *Clinical Cardiology* 30 (March 2007): 125–9.

Korn, Wendy, and Bonnie Siegler. "Miracle Fat-Flushing Foods." *Woman's World*, February 6, 2001.

Krauss, Ronald M., and Darlene M. Dreon. "Low-Density-Lipoprotein Subclasses and Response to a Low-Fat Diet in Healthy Men." *American Journal of Clinical Nutrition* 62, no. 2, S1 (August 1995): 478S–487S.

Kris-Etherton, P.M., Janice Derr, Diane C. Mitchell, Vikkie A. Mustad, Mary E. Russell, Elaine T. McDonnell, Deborah Salabsky and Tomas A. Pearson. "The Role of Fatty Acid Saturation on Plasma Lipids, Lipoproteins, and Apolipoproteins: I. Effects of Whole Food Diets High in Cocoa Butter, Olive Oil, Soybean Oil, Dairy Butter, and Milk Chocolate on the Plasma Lipids of Young Men." *Metabolism* 42, no. 1 (January 1993): 121–9.

Krishman, Supriya, Lynn Rosenberg, Martha Singer, Frank B. Hu, Luc Djoussé, Adrienne Cupples, and Julie R. Palmer. "Glycemic Index, Glycemic Load, and Cereal Fiber Intake and Risk of Type 2 Diabetes in U.S. Black Women." *Archives of Internal Medicine* 167, no. 21 (2007): 2304–9.

Kromhout, Daan. "Serum Cholesterol in Cross-Cultural Perspective: The Seven Countries Study." *Acta Cardiol* 54, no. 3 (June 1999): 155–8.

Kromhout, Daan, Alessandro Menotti, Bennie Bloemberg, Chris Aravanis, Henry Blackburn, Ratko Buzina, Anastasios S. Dontas, Flaminio Fidanza, Simona Giampoli, Annemarie Jansen, Martti Karvonen, Martijn Katan, Aulikki Nissinen, Srecko Nedeljkovic, Juha Pekkanen, Maija Pekkarinen, Sven Punsar, Leena Rasanen, Bozidar Simic, and Hironori Toshima. "Dietary Saturated and trans Fatty Acids and Cholesterol and 25-Year Mortality from Coronary Heart Disease: The Seven Countries Study." *Preventive Medicine* 24, no. 3 (May 1995): 308–15.

Kromhout, Daan, Edward B. Bosschieter, and Cor De Lezenne Coulander. "The Inverse Relation Between Fish Consumption and 20-Year Mortality From Coronary Heart Disease." *New England Journal of Medicine* 312, no. 19 (May 9, 1985): 1205–9.

Kruger, J. "Prevalence of Regular Physical Activity among Adults—United States, 2001 and 2005." *JAMA* 299, no. 1 (2008): 30–2.

Kuriyama, Shinichi, Taichi Shimazu, Kaori Ohmori, Nobutaka Kikuchi, Naoki Nakaya, Yoshikazu Nishino, Yoshitaka Tsubono, and Ichiro Tsuji. "Green Tea Consumption and Mortality in Japan." *JAMA* 296, no. 10 (2006): 1255–65.

Leitzman, Michael F., Yikung Park, Aaron Blair, Rachel Ballard-Barbash, Traci Mouw, Albert R. Hollenbeck, and Arthur Scatzkin. "Physical Activity Recommendations and Decreased Risk of Mortality." *Archives of Internal Medicine* 167, no. 22 (2007): 2453–60.

Lindgren, Frank T., Gerald L. Adamson, Virgie G. Shore, Gary J. Nelson, and Perla C. Schmidt. "Effect of a Salmon Diet on the Distribution of Plasma Lipoproteins and Apolipoproteins in Normolipidemic Adult Men." *Lipids* 26, no. 2 (February 1991): 97–101.

Liu, Simin, JoAnn E. Manson, Meir J. Stampfer, Kathryn M. Rexrode, Frank B. Hu, Eric B. Rimm, Walter C. Willett. "Whole Grain Consumption and Risk of Ischemic Stroke in Women." *JAMA* 284, no. 12 (September 27, 2000): 1534–40.

Ludwig, David S. "Childhood Obesity—The Shape of Things to Come." *New England Journal of Medicine* 357, no. 23 (2007): 2325–7.

Ludwig, David. S. "The Glycemic Index: Physiological Mechanisms Relating to Obesity, Diabetes, and Cardiovascular Disease." *JAMA* 287, no. 18 (May 8, 2002): 2414–23.

Maggio, Marcello, Fulvio Lauretani, Gian Paolo Ceda, Stefania Bandinelli, Shari M.

Ling, E. Jeffrey Metter, Andrea Artoni, Laura Carassale, Anna Cazzato, Graziano

Ceresini, Jack M. Guralnik, Shehzad Basaria, Giorgio Valenti, and Luigi Ferrucci.

"Relationship between Low Levels of Anabolic Hormones and 6-Year Mortality

in Older Men: The Aging in the Chianti Area (InCHIANTI) Study."
Archives of Internal Medicine 167, no.20 (November 12, 2007):2249–54.

Maron, David J. Guo Ping Lu, Nai Sheng Cai, Zong Gui Wu, Yue Hua Li, Hui Chen, Jian Qiu Zhu, Xue Juan Jin, Bert C. Wouters, and Jian Zhao. "Cholesterol-Lowering Effect of a Theaflavin-enriched Green Tea Extract." *Archives of Internal Medicine* 163, no. 12 (June 23, 2003): 1448–53.

McAnlis, G.T., J. McEneny, J. Pearce, and I.S. Young. "Black Tea Consumption Does Not Protect Low Density Lipoprotein from Oxidative Modification." *European Journal of Clinical Nutrition* 52, no. 3 (March 1998): 202–6.

McGee, Daniel, Dwayne Reed, Grant Stemmerman, George Rhoads, Katsuhiko Yano, and Manning Feinleib. "The Relationship of Dietary Fat and Cholesterol to Mortality in 10 Years: The Honolulu Heart Program." *International Journal of Epidemiology* 14, no. 1 (1985): 97–105.

McGill, Jr., Henry C. "The Relationship of Dietary Cholesterol to Serum Cholesterol Concentration and to Atherosclerosis in Man." *American Journal of Clinical Nutrition* 32, no. 12 (1979): 2664–702.

McTigue, Kathleen, Joseph C. Larson, Alice Valoski, Greg Burke, Jane Kotchen, Cora E. Lewis, Marcia L. Stefanick, Linda Van Horn, and Lewis Kuller. "Mortality and Cardiac and Vascular Outcomes in Extremely Obese Women." *JAMA* 296, no. 1 (2006): 79–86.

Menotti, A., H. Blackburn, D. Kromhout, A. Nissinen, F. Fidanza, S. Giampaoli, R. Buzina, I. Mohacek, S. Nedeljkovic, C. Aravanis, and H. Toshima. "Changes in Population

Cholesterol Levels and Coronary Heart Disease Deaths in Seven Countries." *European Heart Journal* 18 (1997): 566–71.

Mitrou, Panagiota N., Victor Kipnis, Anne C. M. Thiébaut, Jill Reedy, Amy F. Subar, Elisabet Wirfält, Andrew Flood, et al. "Mediterranean Dietary Pattern and Prediction of All-Cause Mortality in a U.S. Population: From the Results of the NIH-AARP Diet and Health Study." *Archives of Internal Medicine* 167, no. 22 (2007): 2461–8.

Mellen, Philip B., Sue K. Gao, Mara Z. Vitolins, and David C. Goff. "Deteriorating Habits among Adults with Hypertension." *Archives of Internal Medicine* 168, no. 3 (2008): 308–14.

Mensink, Ronald P., and Martijn B. Katan. "Effect of Dietary Trans Fatty Acids on High-Density and Low-Density Lipoprotein Cholesterol Levels in Healthy Subjects." *New England Journal of Medicine* 323, no. 7 (August 16, 1990): 439–45.

Meriwether, Rebecca A., Jeffrey A. Lee, Augusta Schroeder Lafleur, and Pamela Wiseman. "Physical Activity Counseling." *American Family Physician* 77, no. 8 (April 15, 2008): 1129–36.

Mochari, Heidi. "H is for Higher: Diet Tips for Raising HDL-Cholesterol." *Heart Health Times* 4, no. 2 (Winter 2008): 2.

Mochari, Heidi. "New York City Board of health Bans Trans Fats at Restaurants." *Heart Health Times* 4, no. 1 (Summer 2007): 1–2.

Mosca, Lori. "HDL Raising Drugs: In Search of the Holy Grail?" *Heart Health Times* 4, no. 2 (Winter 2008): 1.

Mosca, Lori. "Red Alert: Updated Prevention Guidelines for Women." *Heart Health Times* 4, no. 1 (Summer 2007): 1.

Mozaffarian, Dariush, Aruna Kamineni, Ronald J. Prineas, and David S. Siscovick. "Metabolic Syndrome and Mortality in Older Adults." *Archives of Internal Medicine* 168, no. 9 (May 12, 2008): 969–78.

Mozaffarian, Dariush, Martijin B. Katan, Alberto Ascherio, Meir J. Stampfer, and Walter C. Willett. "Trans Fatty Acids and Cardiovascular Disease." *New England Journal of Medicine* 354, no. 15 (2006): 1601–12.

Mozaffarian, Dariush, Shiriki K. Kumanyika, Rozenn N. Lemaitre, Jean L. Olson, Gregory L. Burke, David S. Siscovick. "Cereal, Fruit, and Vegetable Fiber Intake and the Risk of Cardiovascular Disease in Elderly Individuals." *JAMA* 289, no. 13 (April 2, 2003): 1659–66.

Mozaffarian, Dariush, W. T. Longstreth Jr., Rozenn N. Lemaitre, Teri A. Manolio, Lewis H. Kuller, Gregory L. Burke, and David S. Siscovick. "Fish Consumption and Stroke Risk." *Cardiology Review* 22, no. 7 (2005): 20–4.

Nambi, Vijay, Byron J. Hoogwerf, and Dennis L. Sprecher. "A Truly Deadly Quartet: Obesity, Hypertension, Hypertriglyceridemia, and Hyperinsulinemia." *Cleveland Clinic Journal of Medicine* 69, no. 2 (December 2002): 985–9.

Nash, Stephen D., and Matthew Westpfal. "Cardiovascular Benefits of Nuts." *American Journal of Cardiology* 95 (April 15, 2005): 963–4.

Nestel, P.J. "Effects of N-3 Fatty Acids on Lipid Metabolism." *Annual Review of Nutrition* 10 (1990): 149-167.

Nestel, Paul J. "How Good is Chocolate?" *American Journal of Clinical Nutrition* 74, no. 5 (November 2001): 563–4.

Nijveldt, Robert J., Els van Nood, Danny EC van Hoorn, Petra G Boelens, Klaske van Norren, and Paul A.M. van Leeuwen. "Flavonoids: A Review of Probable Mechanisms of Action and Potential Applications." *American Journal of Clinical Nutrition* 74, no. 4 (October 2001): 418–25.

NoCarbZone.com. "Glycemic Index vs. Glycemic Load. NoCarbZone.com. http://www.nocarbzone.com/html/ GI_v_GL.html (accessed 04/17/2008).

Paparrigopoulos, Thomas, Elias Tzavellas, Dimitris Karaiskos, and Ioannis Liappas. "The Relationship between Testosterone and Mortality in Men: A Debatable Issue." *Archives of Internal Medicine* 168, no. 3 (2008): 329.

Pereira, Mark A., David R. Jacobs Jr., Linda Van Horn, Martha L. Slattery, Alex I. Kartashov, and David S. Ludwig. "Dairy Consumption, Obesity, and the Insulin Resistance Syndrome in Young Adults: The CARDIA Study." *JAMA* 287, no. 16 (April 24, 2002): 2081–9.

Pietinen, Pirjo, Erkki Vartiainen, Ritva Seppanen, Antti Aro, and Pekka Puska. "Changes in Diet in Finland 1972 to 1992: Impact on Coronary Heart Disease Risk." *Preventive Medicine* 25, no. 6 (November 1996): 243–50.

Pletcher, Mark J., and Robert B. Baron. "Primary Prevention of Cardiovascular Disease in Women: New Guidelines and Emerging Strategies." *Johns Hopkins Advanced Studies in Medicine* 5, no. 8 (2005): 412–9.

Post, Wendy S. "The Metabolic Syndrome: The 'Deadly Quartet.'" *Cardiology Review* 22, no.6 (2005): 32.

Raloff, Janet. "An Apple a Day Keeps the Oncologist Away." Science News Online. http://www.sciencenews.org/sn_ arc97/8_2_97/food.htm (accessed 05/28/2000).

Raloff, Janet. "Berry Good Protection for Aging Brains." Science News Online. http://www.sciencenews.org/sn_arc99/9_18_99/fob2.htm (accessed 05/28/2000).

Raloff, Janet. "Chocolate Hearts: Yummy and Good Medicine?" Science News Online. http://www.sciencenews.org/20000318/bob2.asp (accessed 05/28/2008).

Raloff, Janet. "Grape Juice: Better than Aspirin?" Science News Online. http://www.sciencenews.org/sn_arc97/3_22_97/food.htm (accessed 05/28/2000).

Renaud, Serge, Michel de Lorgeril, Jacques Delaye, Janine Guidellot, Franck Jacquard, Nicole Mamelle, Jean-Louis Martin, Isabelle Monjaud, Patricia Salen, and Paul Toubol. "Cretan Mediterranean Diet for Prevention of Coronary Heart Disease." *American Journal of Clinical Nutrition* 61, no. 6, S1 (June 1995): 1360S–1367S.

RightHealth. "Glycemic Load." RightHealth. http://www.righthealth.com/

Health/glycemic_load/-od-definition_wiki_Glycemic_load-s (accessed 04/17/2008).

Rosmarin, P.C., W.B. Applegate, and G.W. Somes. "Coffee Consumption and Serum Lipids: A Randomized, Crossover Clinical Trial." *American Journal of Medicine* 89, no. 6 (December 1990): 836.

Rousell, Michael A., and Penny Kris-Etherton. "Effects of Lifestyle Interventions on High-Density Lipoprotein Cholesterol Levels." *Journal of Clinical Lipidology* 1, no.1 (2007): 65–73.

Samaha, Frederick, Nayyar Iqbal, Prakash Seshadri, Kethryn L. Chicano, Denise A. Daily, Joyce McGrory, Terrence Williams, Monica Williams, Edward C. Gracely, and Linda

Stern. "A Low-Carbohydrate as Compared with a Low-Fat Diet in Severe Obesity." *New England Journal of Medicine* 348, no. 21 (May 22, 2003): 2074–81.

Sanders, Lisa. "Protein Power: The Myths and Realities of Low-Carb Diets." *Cortlandt Forum*, July 2003.

Schillaci, Giuseppe, Matteo Pirro, Gaetano Vaudo, Fabio Gernelli, and Elmo Mannarino. "The Metabolic Syndrome and Essential Hypertension." *Cardiology Review* 22, no. 6 (2005): 32–4

Schulze, Matthias B., JoAnn E. Manson, David S. Ludwig, Graham A. Colditz, Meir J. Stampfer, Walter C. Willett, and Frank B. Hu. "Sugar-Sweetened Beverages, Weight Gain, and Incidence of Type 2 Diabetes in Young and Middle-Aged Women." *JAMA* 292, no. 8 (2004): 927–34.

Schwartz, Gregory G., and Anders G. Olsson. "The Case for Intensive Stain Therapy After Acute coronary Syndromes." *American Journal of Cardiology* 96, no. 5A (September 5, 2005): 45–53.

Sesso, H.D., J.M. Gaziano, J.E. Buring, and C.H. Hennekens. "Coffee and Tea Intake and the Risk of Myocardial Infarction." *American Journal of Epidemiology* 149, no. 2 (January 15, 1999): 162–7.

Shekelle, Richard B., and Jeremiah Stamler. "Dietary Cholesterol and Ischaemic Heart Disease." *The Lancet* May 27, 1989 (8648): 1177–9.

Shekelle, Richard B., Anne MacMillan, Oglesby Paul, Mark Lepper, Jeremiah Stamler, Shuguey Liu, and William Raynor. "Diet, Serum Cholesterol, and Death From Coronary Heart Disease." *New England Journal of Medicine* 304, no. 2 (January 8, 1981): 65–70.

Simopoulos, Artemis, Helen A. Norman, James E. Gillaspy, and James A. Duke. "Common Purslane: A Source of Omega-3 Fatty Acids and Antioxidants." *Journal of the American College of Nutrition* 1, no. 4 (August 1992): 374–82.

Sjöström, Lars, Anna-Karin Lindroos, Markku Peltonen, Jarl Torgerson, Claude Bouchard, Björn Carlsson, Sven Dahlgren, et al. "Lifestyle, Diabetes, and Cardiovascular Risk Factors 10 Years after Bariatric Surgery." *New England Journal of Medicine* 351, no. 26 (2004): 2683–93.

Southbeach-diet-plan.com. "South Beach Diet and Glycemic Index Food Chart." Southbeach-diet-plan.com. http://www. southbeach-diet-plan.com/glycemicfoodchart.htm (accessed 04/17/2008).

Stamler, Jeremiah, Martha L. Daviglus, Daniel B. Garside, Alan R. Dyer, Philip Greenland, and James D. Neaton. "Relationship of baseline Serum Cholesterol Levels in 3 Large Cohorts of Younger Men to Long-term Coronary, Cardiovascular, and All-Cause Mortality and to Longevity." *JAMA* 284, no.3 (July 19, 2000): 311–8.

Stone, Neil J., and David Saxon. "Approach to Treatment of the Patient with Metabolic Syndrome: Lifestyle Therapy." *American Journal of Cardiology* 96, no. 4A (2005): 15E–21E.

Strandberg, Timo E., Arto Strandberg, Veikko V. Salomaa, Kaisu Pitkälä, Reijo S. Tilvis, and Tatu A. Miettinen. "The Association between Weight Gain Up to Midlife, 30-Year Mortality, and Quality of Life in Older Men." *Archives of Internal Medicine* 167, no. 20 (2007): 2260–1.

"Study Shows Exercise Reduces Mortality." *Healthy Lifestyles for Healthy Aging*, no. 1 (February 2008): 1–2.

Stump, Craig S., James R. Sowers, and Stephen P. Thomson. "Obesity: Are We Prepared to Act?" *JCMS*, Winter 2007, 5–7.

Sugano, Michihiro. "Characteristics of Fats in Japanese Diets and Current Recommendations." *Lipids* 31, S1 (1996): S283–S286.

Sui, Xuemei, Michael J. LaMonte, James N. Laditka, James W. Hardin, Nancy Chase, Steven P. Hooker, and Steven N. Blair. "Cardiorespiratory Fitness and Adiposity as Mortality Predictors in Older Adults." *JAMA* 298, no. 21 (2007): 2507–16.

Svetkey, Laura P., Victor J. Stevens, Phillip J. Brantley, Lawrence J. Appel, Jack F. Hollis, Catherine M. Loria, William M. Vollmer, Christina M. Gullion, Kristine Funk, Pati Smith, Carmen Samuel-Hodge, Valerie Myers, Lillian F. Lien, Daniel Laferriere, Betty Kennedy, Gerald J. Jerome, Fran Heinith, David W. Harsha, Pamela Evans, Thomas P. Erlinger, Arline T. Dalcin, Janelle Coughlin, Jeanne Charleston, Catherine M. Champagne, Alan Bauck, Jamy D. Ard, and Kathleen Aicher. "Comparison of Strategies for Sustaining Weight Loss: The Weight Loss Maintenance Randomized Controlled Test." *JAMA* 299, no. 10 (March 12, 2008): 1139–48.

Tall, Alan. "Does a High Level of HDL Protect Against Atherosclerosis: Insights from Recent Basic and Clinical Studies." *Heart Health Times* 4, no. 2 (Winter 2008): 1–2.

Taubert, Dirk, Renate Roesen, Clara Lehmann, Norma Jung, and Edgar Schömig. "Effects of Low Habitual Cocoa Intake on Blood Pressure and Bioactive Nitric Oxide: A Randomized Controlled Trial." *JAMA* 298, no. 1 (2007): 49–60.

Toshima, Hironori, Yoshinori Koga, Alessandro Menotti, Ancel keys, Henry Blackburn, David R. Jacobs, and Fulvia Seccareccia. "The Seven Countries Study in Japan." *Japanese Heart Journal* 36, no. 2 (March 1995): 179–89.

Trichopoulou, Antonia, Tina Costacou, Christina Bamia, and Dimitros Trichopoulos. "Adherence to a Mediterranean Diet and Survival in a Greek Population." *New England Journal of Medicine* 348, no. 26 (June 26, 2003): 2599–2608.

Tsai, Chung-Jyi, Michael F. Leitzmann, Wlater C. Willett, and Edward L. Giovannucci. "Fruit and Vegetable Consumption and Risk of Cholecystectomy in Women." *American Journal of Medicine* 119 (2006): 760–7.

Tufts University. "Tomato Products Reduce LDL Cholesterol by 13%." Tufts University Health & Nutrition Letter, March 2008. http://www.tuftshealthletter.com/ShowArticle. aspx?rowId=93 (accessed 07/01/2008).

Vigilante, Kevin, and Mary Flynn. *Low-Fat Lies: High-Fat Frauds.* Washington, D.C.: Regnery Publishing, 2000.

Villegas, Raquel, Simin Liu, Yu-Tang Gao, Gong Yang, Honglan Li, Wei Zheng, and Xiao Ou Shu. "Prospective Study of Dietary Carbohydrates, Glycemic Index, Glycemic Load, and Incidence of Type 2 Diabetes Mellitus in Middle-Aged Chinese Women." *Archives in Internal Medicine* 167, no. 21 (2007): 2310–16.

Vogel, R.A. "The Mediterranean Diet and Endothelial Function: Why Some Dietary Fats May be Healthy." *Cleveland Clinic Journal of Medicine* 67, no. 4 (April 2000): 235–6.

Volek, Jeff S., and Eric C. Westman. "Very-Low-Carbohydrate Weight-Loss Diets Revisited." *Cleveland Clinic Journal of Medicine* 69, no.11 (November 2002): 849–62.

Wellberry, Caroline. "Low-Carbohydrate Diet Effective in Women." *American Family Physician* 76, no. 10 (November 15, 2007): 1545–50.

Westman, Eric, and Neil J. Stone. "Is a Low-Carbohydrate Diet the Best Diet for Metabolic Syndrome?" *Internal Medicine News* 40, no. 14 (July 15, 2007):11.

Willcox, Bradley J., D. Craig Willcox, and Makoto Suzuki. *The Okinawa Program: How the World's Longest-Living People Achieve Everlasting Health—And How You Can Too.* New York: Clarkson Potter, 2001.

Winkelmayer, Wolfgang C., Meir J. Stampfer, Walter C. Willett, and Gary C. Curhan. "Habitual Caffeine Intake and the Risk of Hypertension in Women." *JAMA* 294, no. 18 (2005): 2330–5.

Yates, Laurel B., Luc Djoussé, Tobias Kurth, Julie E. Buring, and Michael Gaziano. "Exceptional Longevity in Men: Modifiable Factors Associated with Survival and Function to Age 90 Years." *Archives of Internal Medicine* 168, no. 3 (2008): 284–90.

Zethelius, Bjorn, Liisa Byberg, C. Nicholas Hales, Hans Lithell, and Christina Berne. "Proinsulin Is an Independent Predictor of Coronary Heart Disease: Report From a 27-Year Follow-Up Study." *Circulation* 105, no. 18 (May 7, 2002): 2153–7.

About the Author

Raymond Adamcik, MD, graduated with honors from Rutgers University with a degree in chemistry, attended medical school at the University of Medicine and Dentistry of New Jersey, and completed his post-doctoral training in Loma Linda University Medical Center. He became board-certified in internal medicine in 1981 then went into private practice, which he still maintains in Florida, treating over ten thousand patients in his career.

Dr. Adamcik is a former associate professor of medicine at USC, was affiliated with the renowned Scripps Clinic in San Diego, and has been a sought-after speaker for various pharmaceutical companies due to his expertise in the areas of diet and medication therapy for conditions such as metabolic syndrome and high cholesterol.

For decades, Dr. Adamcik has been actively involved in independent research on dietary treatment methods and has been a major contributor to medical studies on cholesterol. His practice specializes in treating obesity, metabolic syndrome, diabetes, hypertension, elevated cholesterol (utilizing advanced blood analyzing techniques), and other cardiovascular conditions. His medical and dietary recommendations combine extensive research with years of practical experience.

The results of the Globe's Best Diet are proven by global scientific evidence and verified by individual patients' outcomes—including the author himself.

Acknowledgments

First, I have to thank my strongest supporter, my mother, Georgia Adamcik, without whom this work would not have been possible. She has been my right-hand help in the production of this book. Particularly I am thankful for the fabulous recipes that not only has she created for the book, but has also cooked for me with perfection, to my great fortune.

Next, I would like to thank my left-hand assistant, my wife, Susan. Her computer genius has helped me scale the obstacles that were out of my grasp. She had also tolerated my quirky diets over the years and helped in the development of some recipes.

Next, I would like to thank Chris Trionfo for his expertise in the production of my extensive bibliography.

I would also like to thank Holmes Regional Hospital Library for their assistance in procuring many of the obscure articles that were used in research for this publication.

Finally I would like to thank my friends that supplied emotional support, and my children, Ryan and Brandon, that tolerated my many hours of work and research.

Index

A

abdominal obesity, in children, 15
activity levels
  caveman era, 7
  modern day, 14
  post-Industrial Revolution, 8
  recent upturn in, 51
  weight gain and, 19
adherence, to diet, compared to
  compliance, 36
adult diabetes (Type II), 23
affirmations, 34, 80
African Americans/Blacks
  exercise rate, 51
  overweight/obesity rates, 12–13
agriculture, effects of, on eating, 8,
  13
AHA (American Heart Association)
  food pyramid, 7, 8
  guidelines, 6, 8–9
alcohol
  cautions/concerns, 112–113
  pros/cons, 112
  protective effects of, 113, 114
alcoholic spirits
  low source of flavonoids, 110
  protective effects of, 114
almonds, and cholesterol reduction,
  90
Alzheimer's disease
  French diet and, 110
  protective effects of fruit and
    vegetable juices, 110

American Heart Association (AHA)
  food pyramid, 7, 8
  guidelines, 6, 8–9
*American Journal of Clinical
  Nutrition*, 62
Americans
  bread intake, 65–66
  carbohydrate intake, 57
  diabetes rate, 23
  as good patients, 9
  lack of exercise, 14
  laziness, 14–15
  margarine use, 95
  and obesity epidemic, 12
  oils intake, 94
  omega-3 intake, 84
  sugar intake, 57
  and sweet-tasting food, 13
  weight gain patterns, 18
amputations, and diabetes, 23
antibiotics, 9
anti-inflammatories, and omega-3s,
  85–86
antioxidants
  flavonoids and, 107
  in foods in natural state, 61
  fruits as source of, 78
  vegetables as source of, 75
apathy, weight gain and, 17, 22
apples
  flavonoids source of, 79
  glycemic index/load and, 60
Apricot-Dijon Chicken (recipe),
  134–135

arthritis
exercise difficulties, 25
metabolic rates, 25
weight gain and, 19, 25
Atkins, Robert, 10
Atkins diet
and carrots, 60
mentioned, 1, 2
problems with, 68, 105, 125–126
Atkins-type diets
and butter, 67
and cholesterol level, 68, 105
problems with, 68

B

bad advice, low-fat diet, 15–16
bad cholesterol (LDL)
margarine, negative effects on, 96
nuts, positive effects on, 90
tomatoes, positive effects on, 74
bad foods, say "no" to, 34, 35
Balsamic Vinaigrette (recipe), 138
bariatric surgeries, obesity
treatments, 119–120
beans
Green Beans, 142
Green Beans and Tomatoes, 142
Minestrone, 131
Vegetarian Chili, 130
beef
and Atkins diet, 10
and Cretan diet, 56
fat, 11
food with high cholesterol
content, 117
and Greek diet, 10
politics of not recommending
eating, 57
beer
and cardio-metabolic syndrome,
115

low source of flavonoids, 110
protective effects of, 114
biking, 43
binge-eating, 36
black tea, 108, 109
blindness, and diabetes, 23, 24
blood pressure
alcohol use and, 113
and cardio-metabolic syndrome,
29
chocolate, positive effects on, 108
diastolic, 22
diet colas and, 65
hypertension, 30, 37, 71
impact of bariatric surgery on,
119
systolic, 22
and weight, 22
blood sugar
and cardio-metabolic syndrome,
29
hunger triggers, 70, 78
insulin and, 69, 70
olive oil, positive effects on, 92
recommended level, 28
blueberries, and flavonoids, 79
BMI (Body Mass Indicator)
defined, 20, 22
table, 21*t*
bok choy, as protection against
cancer, 74
boredom, reason to eat, 35
Boston Market, healthier choice, 99
bowling, as exercise, 43
breakfast
high glycemic index/load and, 65
importance of, 54, 64–65
breast cancer
and alcohol use, 113
exercise as protection against, 37,
46

flavonoids as protection against, 107

high glycemic index and, 59–60

and obesity, 24

omega-3s as protection against, 86

broccoli, as protection against cancer, 74

Burger King

chicken sandwich, trans-fatty acid content, 99*t*

french fries, trans-fatty acid content, 99*t*

butter

and Atkins-type diet, 67

compared to margarine, 95–96

consumer preference for, 11

dangerous, 94

and French diet, 10, 100

olive oil as alternative to, 98

C

cabbage soup diet, 1, 41, 42

cabernet sauvignon, source of flavonoids, 109

calcium, 103

calories

and exercise, 47

in fats, 15, 82

intake compared to expenditure, 38

negative calories, 38

and processed foods, 13

reasonable cutting of, 41

and weight training, 48–51

camellia sinensis (tea plant), 109

cancer

exercise as protection against, 37

flavonoids as protection against, 107

fruits as protection against, 78

and obesity, 24

vegetables as protection against, 74

See also specific types

canola oil

recommended, 93, 94

source of omega-3s, 93

carbohydrates

differentiating good from bad, 59, 65–66, 67

high-carbohydrate diet, 8–9

medical term for sugars, 58

and processed foods, 13

carbonated beverages, high glycemic index food, 59

cardio-metabolic syndrome

beer drinking and, 115

causes of, 30

compared to cigarette smoking, 31

defined, 17–18

diagnosis criteria, 29

fish oil, positive effects on, 87

impact of bariatric surgery on, 119

lack of symptoms early on, 31

Mediterranean diet as protection against, 91

prevalence of, 29

reversal of, 31

and risk of dying, 31

screening, 29–30

cardiovascular diseases

flavonoids as protection against, 107

vegetables as protection against, 74

cardiovascular system

and diabetes, 23–24

and obesity, 22

carrots, glycemic index/load and, 60

catechin (flavonoid), 109

cathartics, as weight loss tool, 39
cautions/concerns
    alcohol use, 112–113
    fasting, 38
    frying foods, 99–100
    "no cholesterol" labels, 116
    scales, 40–41
caveman diet, 6–8
cervical cancer, and obesity, 24
change of environment, as weight
    loss tool, 35
cheese
    cottage, low in saturated fats, 104
    and Cretan diet, 56
    decision to enjoy, 104
    food with high cholesterol
        content, 117
    Swiss, low in saturated fats, 104
cheese recipes
    Escarole and Meatball Soup,
        140–141
    Greek Salad, 128
    Minestrone, 131
    Roasted Tomato Appetizer, 137
    Wife's Salad, 129
chicken
    food with high cholesterol
        content, 117
    recipes. See poultry recipes
children
    and abdominal obesity, 15
    and diabetes, 23
    lack of exercise, 15
    playing with, as exercise, 43
Chinese diet, 67
chocolate
    and blood pressure reduction,
        108
    and death rate, 108
chocolate, dark
    as guilty pleasure, 111
    source of flavonoids, 108

cholesterol intake, pros/cons,
    117–118
cholesterol levels
    and Atkins-type diets, 68, 105
    bad cholesterol (LDL). See bad
        cholesterol (LDL)
    fat reduction and, 104–105
    good cholesterol (HDL). See
        good cholesterol (HDL)
    and low-fat diet, 15
    medication to control, 104
    nuts, positive effects on, 90
    olive oil, positive effects on, 92
    omega-3, positive effects on, 85
    and saturated fats, 116
    testing, 28, 118
    and trans-fatty acids, 116
    vegetables, positive effects on, 74
cigarettes. See smoking
Cinnabon, trans-fatty acid content,
    99t
cirrhosis, and obesity, 24
Citrus Salad (recipe), 128
clams, food with high cholesterol
    content, 117
coconut oil, dangerous, 94
coffee, regular compared to decaf,
    108
cola, compared to natural juices, 65
colon cancer
    exercise as protection against, 46
    high glycemic index and, 60
    and obesity, 24
colorectal cancer, vegetables as
    protection against, 74
compliance, with diet, compared to
    adherence, 36
control, of eating habits, 35
cooking
    fish, 87
    meat, 103
    recipes. See recipes

vegetables, 76
corn oil, less desirable, 93
coronary disease
    alcohol use and, 112
    diet cause, 9
    geographic differences in rate of, 9
    nurses' health study, 84–85, 93
    projected increase in, 15
    weight gain and, 17
cottage cheese
    low glycemic index/load, 65
    low in saturated fats, 104
cottonseed oil, less desirable, 93
Creole Scallops (recipe), 139–140
Cretan diet
    compared to Globe's Best Diet, 84
    and dairy products, 56
    and fish, 56
    and flavonoids, 109
    and fruits, 80
    as ideal, 55, 57, 78
    and nuts, 56
    and olive oil, 56, 57, 91, 92
    and trans-fatty acids, 100
    typical daily intake, 56*t*
cross-country ski machines, 44
Cucumber Dill Sauce (recipe), 141

D

dairy fat, 11
dairy products
    in Cretan diet, 56
    low glycemic index/load and, 65
    provide fullness, 104
    source of calcium, 103
    source of vitamin D, 103
dancing, as exercise, 43
dark beer, source of flavonoids, 110
DART diet, 90

DASH diet, 73–74
death
    early, and diabetes, 23
    obesity and, 26
    physical inertia cause, 37, 46
    rate, and chocolate, 108
    weight gain and risk of, 19–20
decaf coffee, and increased risk of heart attack, 108
denial, weight gain and, 18
depression
    exercise as improvement for, 46
    weight gain and, 19
diabetes
    adult diabetes (Type II), 23
    and amputations, 23
    and blindness, 23, 24
    and cardiovascular system, 23–24
    and children, 23, 69
    and early death, 23
    exercise as protection against, 37, 45–46
    and heart attacks, 5, 23
    heredity effects on, 30
    high glycemic index foods and, 59, 66
    and high vegetable and fruit intake, 75
    impact of bariatric surgery on, 119
    and kidney failure, 23
    and lifestyle changes, 24
    and male impotency, 23
    nuts as protection against, 90
    and obesity, 22
    rate of, in America, 23
    rice consumption and, 67
    and strokes, 23
    Type I (juvenile diabetes), 23, 69
    Type II (adult diabetes), 23
    weight gain and, 17
    whole grain products and, 66

diabetes mellitus, 22, 69
diastolic blood pressure, 22
diets
    Atkins, 1, 2, 60, 68, 105, 125–126
    Atkins-type, 68, 105
    cabbage soup, 1, 41, 42
    caveman, 6–8
    Chinese, 67
    compared to lifestyle changes, 3
    Cretan. *See* Cretan diet
    DART, 90
    DASH, 73–74
    Eskimo, 10, 83
    experimental, 8
    fad, 1, 3
    failings of, 1, 2, 3
    Finland, 73, 105
    French, 10, 100, 110
    grapefruit, 1
    Greek, 10, 100, 109
    high-carbohydrate, 2, 8–9, 27–28, 34, 57, 70
    high-fat, 10, 56–57, 67–68, 109
    high-sugar, 66
    history of, 6
    Japanese, 10, 53, 83–84, 93, 109, 117
    long-term health effects, 2, 3
    low-carbohydrate, 10, 67–68
    low-fat. *See* low-fat diets
    Mediterranean, 84, 90, 91. *See also* Cretan diet
    myths, 55–56, 89
    Ornish, 10
    Pritkin, 10, 27–28
    protein, 10
    sample, Globe's Best, 121–123
    short-term results, 2
    as short-term treatments, 4
    soup, 1
    South Beach, 1
    starvation, 2
    three-day, 1
    Weight Watchers, 54
    wine-only, 1
    Zone, 67
discipline, and weight loss, 4, 33, 34
disorders, binge-eating, 36
diuretics, as weight loss tool, 39
dog walking, as exercise, 43
dressings, salad
    Balsamic Vinaigrette, 138
    Garlic-Dijon Vinaigrette, 138
    Simple Vinaigrette Dressing, 138

E

eating
    breakfast, 54, 64–65
    habits, 8, 35, 53, 54
    meal frequency, 53–54
    reasons, 35
    a rich and pleasurable experience, 126
    See also diets; foods
edema, 26
eggs
    food with high cholesterol content, 117
    pros/cons, 116–117, 118
elderly
    exercise, positive effects on, 38
    weight training, positive effects on, 50–51
electronic entertainment, as exercise replacement, 15
elliptical machines, 44
emotional turmoil, and diet changes, 35
Empatic (medication), and weight loss, 120
endorphins, and exercise, 46

endurance, exercise as improvement of, 37–38
energy levels
    diminished with weight gain, 19
    exercise, positive effects on, 34, 37
    improved with treatment, 119
epidemic, obesity, 8, 12–16
Escarole and Meatball Soup (recipe), 140
Eskimo diet
    and lack of heart problems, 10, 83
    and use of omega-3s, 83
esophageal cancer, and obesity, 24
essential nutrients
    combined with sugars, 58
    described, 86
    number of, 1, 2
    and processed foods, 8
Europeans, and walking, 14
exercise
    benefits, 34, 37–38, 45–46
    calories burned, 47
    in caveman era, 7
    equipment, 38, 43, 44, 45, 47
    excuses for lack of, 44–45
    health effects of, 37–38, 45–46
    lack of, prevalence of, 37
    moderate compared to vigorous, 47
    modern day, 14
    playing with children, 43
    post-Industrial Revolution, 8
    rates, 51
    recommended amount of, 46–47
    sample workout program, 47, 48t
    variety of, 47
    vigorous compared to moderate, 47
    weight training, 48–51
    weight-bearing, 45

expectations, of weight loss, 4
experimental diet, 8

F
fad diets, 1, 3
fast foods
    "fat food" restaurants, 125
    trans-fatty acids and, 99t
fasting, cautions/concerns of, 38
fat loss, compared to fluid loss, 39
fatal fats, 106
fatigue, progressive daytime, and weight gain, 24–25
fats
    as body requirement, 1
    and calories, 15, 82
    diversity of, 81, 82
    excess sugar, stored as, 70
    fatal fats, 106
    healthy compared to lethal, 81
    monosaturated, 90, 92, 105
    nuts, as source of, 82
    as protection against heart attacks, 81
    reduction, and cholesterol level, 104–105
    restrictions, combined with protein reduction, 57
    saturated fats, 101, 102t–103t, 106, 116
    vegetable compared to dairy and animal, 11
    and weight loss, 81–82
    See also specific types
fattening sugars, compared to nutritious sugars, 58–59
fiber
    processed foods and, 61
    vegetables as source of, 74
Finland
    diet, 105

health ranking, 73
fish
   in Cretan diet, 56
   flat compared to fat, 86
   food with high cholesterol
     content, 117
   preparation of, 87
   as protection against strokes, 84
   source of omega-3s, 83, 86–87
fish oil
   capsules, alternative to eating
     fish, 87
   liquid, alternative to capsules, 87
   positive effects on cardio-
     metabolic syndrome, 87
fishing, as exercise, 43
flavonoids
   benefits, 107, 110
   and Cretan diet, 109
   described, 7, 107
   and processed foods, 8
   sources of, 79, 107–108, 111*t*
flax oil
   recommended, 93, 94
   source of omega-3s, 93
flaxseed, source of omega-3s, 90
Fleishmann's margarine, trans-free
  brand, 98
fluid loss, compared to fat loss, 39
food preparation. *See* cooking;
  recipes
food pyramid (AHA), 7, 8
food shopping
   overview, 106
   foods to avoid, 106
   fruits and vegetables, 75–76, 79
   with a list, 35
   meats, 103
   and "no cholesterol" label, 116
   nuts, 91
   processed foods, 98
foods

   with high cholesterol content,
     117*t*
   with high glycemic index, 59–60,
     64
   with high glycemic loads, 67
   natural state benefits, 61
   processed. *See* processed foods
   white in color, 61
   See also specific types
French diet
   and lack of heart problems, 10
   low trans-fatty acid intake, 100
   and reduction in Alzheimer's
     disease, 110
French paradox, 10, 100, 110
Fresh Fruit Salad (recipe), 127
Frisbee, as exercise, 43
fructose (fruit sugar/natural sugar),
  58, 69, 78, 114
fruit recipes
   Citrus Salad, 128
   Fresh Fruit Salad, 127
   Mango Salsa, 133
   Mango-Avocado Salsa, 133
   Mango-Cucumber Salsa, 134
   Orange Chicken, 135
fruit sugar (fructose), 58, 69, 78,
  114
fruits
   antioxidants, source of, 78
   benefits, 78–79
   colorful skins, 79, 107
   described, 78
   and diabetes, 75
   diversity of, 79–80
   juices, 111
   and mental health, 78
   minerals, source of, 78
   recommended servings, 80
   year-round availability, 79
   See also specific types
frying, cautions/concerns, 99–100

G

gallbladder attacks, and obesity, 25
garlic, as protection against cancer,
74
Garlic-Dijon Vinaigrette (recipe),
138
gastric banding, obesity treatment,
119
gastric bypass surgery, obesity
treatment, 119
gastro-esophageal reflux (GERD),
25
gastrointestinal system, and weight
gain, 25
gastrointestinal system cancers
flavonoids as protection against,
107
fruits as protection against, 78
gathering, method for obtaining
food, 6, 7
Gatorade, compared to natural
juices, 65
genetics, 30, 104, 118
GERD (gastro-esophageal reflux),
25
glucose (pure sugar), 59
glycemic index
described, 59
examples of, 62*t*–64*t*
See also high glycemic index foods
glycemic load
described, 60
examples of, 62*t*–64*t*
See also low glycemic index/load
foods
goals, realistic for weight loss, 4
good cholesterol (HDL)
bariatric surgery, impact on, 119
and cardio-metabolic syndrome,
29

heredity effects on low HDL, 30
high glycemic load and, 66
insulin levels and, 71
margarine, negative effects on, 96
omega-3, positive effects on, 85
recommended level, 28
gout, and weight gain, 25
grape juice, purple, benefits, 110
grapefruit diet, 1
grapes, varied levels of flavonoids,
110–111
Greek diet
and flavonoids, 109
and heart problems, 10
low in trans-fatty acids, 100
Greek Salad (recipe), 128
Green Beans and Tomatoes (recipe),
142
Green Beans (recipe), 142
green tea
benefits, 109
as guilty pleasure, 111
Greens (recipe), 129
Grilled Sweet Potatoes (recipe), 140
guilty pleasures, 111
gyms, for exercise, 43–44

H

habits
eating, 8, 35, 53, 54
healthy behaviors and, 34
hara hachi bu (eating principle), 53
HDL (good cholesterol). *See* good
cholesterol (HDL)
healthy behaviors, and habits, 34
heart attacks
decaf coffee and, 108
and diabetes, 23
diet cause, 9
exercise as protection against, 37
and fats, 81

geographic differences in rate of, 9
high-sugar diet and, 66
omega-3s as protection against, 84
heart disease. *See* coronary disease
heart irregularities, fatal, and weight gain, 25
Herb-Roasted Chicken (recipe), 135–136
heredity
and blood cholesterol, 104, 118
and cardio-metabolic syndrome, 30
and diabetes, 30
high glycemic index foods
breakfast and, 64
and breast cancer, 59–60
and colon cancer, 60
described, 59–60
and diabetes, 6659
nuts as substitute for, 91
high glycemic loads
examples of foods with, 67
and good cholesterol (HDL), 66
high-carbohydrate diets, 2, 8–9, 27–28, 39, 57, 70
high-fat diets, 10, 56–57, 67–68, 109
high-sugar diets, 66
high-sugar food items, 69, 70
Hispanics, overweight rate/obesity rates, 12–13
home gym equipment, 45
hormonal and reproductive systems, obesity and, 26
household chores, as exercise, 43
hunger
avoidance of, 53
nuts as suppresser of, 90
processed foods and, 61
triggers, 70

hunting, method of obtaining food, 6, 7
hydrogenation, partial, 95
hypertension (elevated blood pressure)
exercise as protection against, 37
heredity effects on, 30
insulin levels and, 71
hypoglycemia, 82

I
identity, mind generated, 32, 41, 51, 126
impotency (male)
and diabetes, 23
and obesity, 26
industry, effects of, on eating habits, 8
insulin, defined, 69
insulin levels
beer and, 114–115
blood sugar and, 69, 70
cholesterol and, 71
effects of, 70, 71
exercise reduction and, 47
high glycemic index and, 59
hypertension and, 71
recommended, 28
insulin resistance, saturated fats cause, 101
International Table of Glycemic Index and Glycemic Load Values: 2002, 62

J
Japanese diet
eating habits, 53
and eggs, 117
and lack of heart problems, 10, 83–84
and soybean oil, 93

and teas, 109
and use of omega-3s, 83–84
jobs, as physical activity, 14
joint pressure, weight gain and, 19,
  25
juices
  fruit juices, 110, 111
  purple grape juice, 110
  vegetable juices, 111

K

KFC biscuit, trans-fatty acid
  content, 99*t*
kidney cancer, and obesity, 24
kidney failure, and diabetes, 23
kielbasa, turkey, Lentil, Turkey
  Kielbasa Stew, 132

L

lard, dangerous, 94
LDL (bad cholesterol). *See* bad
  cholesterol (LDL)
legumes, source of protein, 130
Lentil, Turkey Kielbasa Stew
  (recipe), 132
lettuce, as protection against cancer,
  74
lifestyle changes
  bariatric surgery and, 120
  benefits, 31
  compared to diets, 3
  diabetes and, 24
  livable changes, 41
  mind and, 33
  motivations for, 18, 51
  as opportunities, 36
  physician recommended
    compared to self recommended,
    36
lipids test, 29, 30

liquid meal replacements, and
  weight loss, 99
liver problems, and obesity, 24
lobster, food with high cholesterol
  content, 117
Long John Silver fish, trans-fatty
  acid content, 99*t*
low glycemic index/load foods
  dairy products, 65
  described, 60
  fruits, 78
  nuts, 65
  whole grain products, 65
low-carbohydrate diets
  Atkins diet, 10
  compared to low-fat diets, 67, 68
low-fat diets
  author's experience with, 27–28
  as bad advice, 15–16
  and cholesterol level, 15
  compared to low-carbohydrate
    diets, 67, 68
  compared to Mediterranean diets,
    91
  guilt and, 104, 106
  medical profession
    recommendation, 9–10, 15–16
  myth of, 55–56, 71
  as protection against osteoporosis,
    82
  and protein deficiency, 2, 39
lung cancer
  flavonoids as protection against,
    107
  fruits as protection against, 78
lycopene, 74
Lyon heart study, 84, 93

M

macadamia nuts, benefits, 90
male impotency, 23, 26

maltose (malt-derived sugar), 58, 69, 114–115
Mango Salsa (recipe), 133
Mango-Avocado Salsa (recipe), 133
Mango-Cucumber Salsa (recipe), 134
margarine
    compared to butter, 95–96
    and increased cardiovascular risk, 96
    replacement for butter, 11
    risks associated with, 95–96
    trans-free brands, 98
McDonald's
    chicken nuggets, trans-fatty acid content, 99t
    french fries, trans-fatty acid content, 99t
meal frequency, 53–54
meal plans, Globe's Best Diet, 121–123
Meat Loaf (recipe), 134
meat products, provide fullness, 104
meat recipe, Meat Loaf, 134
medication
    for cholesterol reduction, 104, 120
    and low-fat diets, 9–10, 15–16
    for weight loss, 120
medicine, history of, 9–11
Mediterranean countries, health ranking, 73
Mediterranean diet
    and cardio-metabolic syndrome, 91
    compared to Globe's Best Diet, 84, 90
    compared to typical low-fat diet, 91
    See also Cretan diet
men
    and alcohol intake, 113

calories burned exercising, 42
cardio-metabolic syndrome factors, 29
exercise rate, 51
impotency causes, 23, 26
obesity rate, 12
premature deaths, 26
and prostate cancer, 24, 74
and weight lifting, 48–49
mental health
    exercise, positive effects on, 37–38
    fruits, positive effets on, 78
merlot, source of flavonoids, 109
metabolic rate, 3, 4, 49, 54
metabolic syndrome, 27
    See also cardio-metabolic syndrome
metformin (medication), and weight loss, 120
milk, whole, food with high cholesterol content, 117
mind
    and identity, 32, 41, 51, 126
    and lifestyle changes, 33
minerals
    as body requirement, 1
    fruits as source of, 78
    and processed foods, 8
    vegetables as source of, 75
Minestrone (recipe), 131
monosaturated fat, 90, 92, 105
motivation, for weight loss, 4, 18, 33
mouth cancer, vegetables as protection against, 74
muscle
    defined, 3
    loss of, 2–3, 4, 39, 49
muscle mass, statistics, 49
myths
    diets, 55–56

nuts, 89

N

National Weight Registry (study), 42

natural beverages, examples of, 65

natural sugar (fructose), 58, 69, 78, 114

negative calories, 38

"no," to bad foods, 34, 35

"no cholesterol" labels, cautions/concerns, 116

normal weight, BMI indicator, 22

nurses' health study

  fish intake and heart disease, 84–85

  flax intake and heart disease, 93

nutritious sugars, compared to fattening sugars, 58–59

nuts

  benefits, 89–90, 91

  and cholesterol reduction, 90

  in Cretan diet, 56

  as fat source, 82

  high glycemic index foods substitute, 91

  low glycemic load, 65

  myths about, 89

  olive oil substitute, 91

  source of omega-3s, 83, 87

  and weight loss, 89

O

oat bran, for cholesterol reduction, 65

obesity

  alternative treatments for, 119–120

  and cancer, 24

  and cardiovascular system, 22

  in children, 15

  and cirrhosis, 24

  consequences/complications of, 17–26

  and death, 26

  and depression, 19

  and diabetes, 22

  and eating habits, 54

  and edema, 26

  as epidemic, 8, 12–16

  and gallbladder attacks, 25

  and gastrointestinal problems, 25

  and hormonal and reproductive systems, 26

  and impotency, 26

  and liver problems, 24

  and meal frequency, 54

  and phlebitis (blood clots), 26

  psychological effects of, 26

  rate in America, 12–13

  as result of fad diets, 3

  social effects of, 17, 26

oils

  dangerous kinds, 94

  less desirable kinds, 93

  recommended kinds, 93, 94

  See also fats; *specific types*

olive oil

  as alternative to margarine and butter, 98

  benefits, 92–93

  in Cretan diet, 56, 57, 91, 92

  in Greek diet, 10

  nuts, as substitute, 91

  recommended, 93, 94

omega-3s (omega-3 fats)

  benefits, 83–86

  described, 83

  effect on triglycerides, 87

  fish oil capsules, 87–88

  fish oil liquid, 87

  in Japanese diet, 83–84

  and pregnant women, 86

recommended intake, 84–85, 87
saturated fats substitute, 105
sources of, 83, 85–87, 93
onions, as protection against cancer,
74
Orange Chicken (recipe), 135
Ornish diet, 10
osteoporosis
exercise as protection against, 38,
45
and vitamin D deficiency, 106
Overeaters Anonymous, 35
overweight
BMI indicator, 22
rate, in America, 12
oxygen deficiency, and weight gain,
25

P

palm oil, dangerous, 94
pancreatic cancer, and obesity, 24
partial hydrogenation, 95
pasta, glycemic index/load and, 60
patience, in weight loss effort, 33, 34
peanut oil, less desirable, 93
pecans, benefits, 90
pedometer, step counting, 43
persistence, in weight loss effort, 33,
34–35
Phen-Phen (medication), and weight
loss, 120
phlebitis (blood clots), 26
physical activity. See exercise
physician recommended lifestyle
changes, 36
physicians' health study
and alcohol use, 114
and nuts intake, 90
ping pong, as exercise, 43
pinot noir, source of flavonoids, 109
pistachios, benefits, 90

pizza, pros/cons, 65
plant oils, pros/cons, 93–94
playing with children, as exercise, 43
politics, cause of low-fat
recommendation, 57
popcorn, poor snack choice, 65
potassium, benefits, 74–75
potatoes, high glycemic index/load
food, 59, 65
poultry recipes
Apricot-Dijon Chicken, 134–135
Escarole and Meatball Soup,
140–141
Herb-Roasted Chicken, 135–136
Lentil, Turkey Kielbasa Stew, 132
Meat Loaf, 134
Orange Chicken, 135
pregnant women, and omega-3s, 86
pretzels, poor snack choice, 65
Pritkin diet, 10, 27–28
processed foods
additives in, 13–14
avoidance of, 98
calories and, 13
carbohydrates and, 13
as cheap choices, 13
current era of, 8
disadvantages of, 61
essential nutrients and, 8
and hunger, 61
margarine, 95
minerals and, 8
processed meats compared to red
meat, 103
and saturated fat content, 103
and taste-bud poisoning, 79
Promise margarine, trans-free brand,
98
prostate cancer
and obesity, 24
tomatoes as protection against,
74

protein diet, 10
proteins
  as body requirement, 1
  deficiency of, 2, 3
  vegetables as source of, 75
Prozac, 36
psychological
  changes, 33
  effects of obesity, 26
pure sugar (glucose), 59
purple grape juice, benefits, 110

Q

quercetin (flavonoid), 109
quick fix, for weight problems, 1, 37

R

racquetball, 47
raisins, high glycemic index/load
  and, 65
realistic goals, weight loss, 4
recipes
  Apricot-Dijon Chicken, 134–135
  Balsamic Vinaigrette, 138
  Citrus Salad, 128
  Creole Scallops, 139–140
  Cucumber Dill Sauce, 141
  Escarole and Meatball Soup,
    140–141
  Fresh Fruit Salad, 127
  Garlic-Dijon Vinaigrette, 138
  Greek Salad, 128
  Green Beans, 142
  Green Beans and Tomatoes, 142
  Greens, 129
  Grilled Sweet Potatoes, 140
  Herb-Roasted Chicken, 135–136
  Lentil, Turkey Kielbasa Stew, 132
  Mango Salsa, 133
  Mango-Avocado Salsa, 133
  Mango-Cucumber Salsa, 134

  Meat Loaf, 134
  Minestrone, 131
  Orange Chicken, 135
  Roasted Asparagus, 142
  Roasted Red Pepper Dip, 136
  Roasted Red Peppers, 136
  Roasted Tomato Appetizer, 137
  Shrimp Creole, 139
  Simple Vinaigrette Dressing, 138
  Smothered Okra and Tomatoes,
    143
  Tomato Salsa, 141
  Vegetable Salad with Brown Rice,
    137
  Vegetarian Chili, 130
  Wife's Salad, 129
  Zucchini and Yellow Summer
    Squash, 129
red meat, as compared to processed
  meats, 103
red wine
  as guilty pleasure, 111
  source of flavonoids, 109–110
reproductive and hormonal systems,
  obesity and, 26
reservatrol (flavonoid), 110
restaurant food, and trans-fatty
  acids, 98
rice
  diabetes and, 67
  high glycemic index food, 59
rice recipe, Vegetable Salad with
  Brown Rice, 137
Roasted Asparagus (recipe), 142
Roasted Red Pepper Dip (recipe),
  136
Roasted Red Peppers (recipe), 136
Roasted Tomato Appetizer (recipe),
  137
rollerblading, 43
rowing equipment, 44
rutin (flavonoid), 110

S

safflower, less desirable, 93
sailing, as exercise, 43
salad dressings
    Balsamic Vinaigrette, 138
    Garlic-Dijon Vinaigrette, 138
    Simple Vinaigrette Dressing, 138
salt, reduction in diet, 79
sample diet, meal plans, 121–123
sashimi, source of omega-3s, 87
saturated fats
    cautions/concerns of, 101
    and cholesterol level, 116
    contradictory effects of, 106
    sources of, 102t–103t
sauna, as weight loss tool, 39
say "no," to bad foods, 34, 35
scales, cautions, 40–41
seafood recipes
    Creole Scallops, 139–140
    Shrimp Creole, 139
self-esteem, obesity and, 26
self-worth, 17, 33, 126
sesame oil, less desirable, 93
seven-country study
    animal fats and heart disease link, 93
    and coronary disease, 15
    described, 9
    and effects of saturated fat, 95, 101
    and fats, 11
    and flavonoids, 79, 107
    and Greek diet, 100
    and vegetables, 73
shrimp
    food with high cholesterol content, 117
    pros/cons, 117
    Shrimp Creole, 139

Shrimp Creole (recipe), 139
Simple Vinaigrette Dressing (recipe), 138
sleep apnea, and weight gain, 24
sleeplessness, and weight gain, 24
smoking
    compared to cardio-metabolic syndrome, 31
    compared to weight gain, 12
Smothered Okra and Tomatoes (recipe), 143
snacks, nutritious
    to avoid hunger, 35
    carrots and celery, 76
    fruits, 79, 80
    importance of, 54
    nuts, 90, 91
social effects, of obesity, 17, 26
social prejudice, obesity and, 26
soup diet, 1
South Beach diet, 1
soybean oil
    recommended, 93, 94
    source of omega-3s, 93
soybeans, benefits, 76
spinach, Popeye's secret weapon, 73
starvation diet, 2
statements of desirable intentions, 34, 80
stomach cancer, vegetables as protection against, 74
stress
    and diet changes, 35
    exercise, positive effects on, 37, 46
strokes
    and alcohol use, 114
    and diabetes, 23
    exercise as protection against, 37
    fish as protection against, 84
    high-sugar diet and, 66

vegetables as protection against, 74

whole grain products as protection against, 65, 66

sucrose (table sugar), 58, 69

sugar
  and cholesterol, 71
  defined, 58
  excess stored as fat, 70
  fattening sugars, 58–59
  forms of, 69
  fructose, 58, 69, 78, 114
  glucose, 59
  high-sugar diets, 66
  and low glycemic index foods, 60
  maltose, 58, 69, 114–115
  nutritious sugars, 58–59
  in processed foods, 13, 61
  source of fiber, 57
  sucrose, 58, 69
  and triglyceride production, 71
  types of, 67, 114

sunflower oil, less desirable, 93

sushi, source of omega-3s, 87

sweet potatoes, benefits, 76

swimming, 43

syndrome X, 27
  See also cardio-metabolic syndrome

systolic pressure, 22

T

table sugar (sucrose), 58, 69

tai chi, as exercise, 43

taste
  fish, 83
  fruits, 79
  improving, 76
  salt reduction, 79

teas
  benefits, 109

source of flavonoids, 108

theaflavin (flavonoid), 109

three-day diet, 1

tofu, benefits, 76

Tomato Salsa (recipe), 141

tomatoes
  and flavonoids, 79
  as protection against prostate cancer, 74

toxins, 34

trans-fatty acids, 11
  average daily intake, 96
  and cholesterol, 116
  and Cretan diet, 100
  and fast food restaurants, 99*t*
  intake reduction, 100
  negative effects of, 96
  as poison, 11, 95
  processed foods and, 13
  and restaurant food, 98
  sources of, 97*t*

trans-free brands, 98

treadmills, 38, 43, 44, 45, 47

triglycerides
  and cardio-metabolic syndrome, 29
  defined, 70
  effect on coronary arteries, 70–71
  heredity effects on, 30
  insulin and, 70
  and margarine, 96
  omega-3, positive effects on, 85
  recommended level, 28

turkey. *See* poultry recipes

Type I diabetes (juvenile diabetes), 23, 69

Type II diabetes (adult diabetes), 23

U

underweight, BMI indicator, 22

urinary system cancers

flavonoids as protection against, 107

fruits as protection against, 78

USDA (U.S. Department of Agriculture), recommendations, 7

uterine cancer, and obesity, 24

V

vegetable fat, 11

vegetable phobia, 73

vegetable recipes

Cucumber Dill Sauce, 141

Escarole and Meatball Soup, 140–141

Greek Salad, 128

Green Beans, 142

Green Beans and Tomatoes, 142

Greens, 129

Grilled Sweet Potatoes, 140

Lentil, Turkey Kielbasa Stew, 132

Mango-Cucumber Salsa, 134

Minestrone, 131

Roasted Asparagus, 142

Roasted Red Pepper Dip, 136

Roasted Red Peppers, 136

Roasted Tomato Appetizer, 137

Smothered Okra and Tomatoes, 143

Tomato Salsa, 141

Vegetable Salad with Brown Rice, 137

Vegetarian Chili, 130

Wife's Salad, 129

Zucchini and Yellow Summer Squash, 129

Vegetable Salad with Brown Rice (recipe), 137

vegetables

benefits, 73, 74

childhood tastes and, 75

colorful skins, 107

and diabetes, 75

juices, 111

recommended servings, 77

source of antioxidants, 75

source of minerals, 75

sources of fiber, 74

See also specific types

Vegetarian Chili (recipe), 130

vertical banded gastroplasty, obesity treatment, 119

vitamin B, deficiency, 2

vitamin B-12, 75

vitamin C, deficiency, 2

vitamin D

dairy products as source of, 103

deficiency, 2, 106

vitamins

as body requirement, 1

dairy products, as source of, 103

deficiencies, 2

fruits as source of, 78

processed foods and, 8, 61

vegetables as source of, 75

W

waist circumference, and cardio-metabolic syndrome, 29

walking

alternatives to, 43

and calorie burning, 42

dog walking, 43

as weight loss tool, 42–43

walnuts, source of omega-3s, 90

water, fruits as source of, 78

water depletion, cautions against, 40

weight

and blood pressure, 22

normal, and BMI indicator, 22

weight gain

and apathy, 17, 22

compared to smoking, 12

consequences/complications of,
17, 19–26
and denial, 18
and depression, 19
and diabetes, 17
and gastrointestinal system, 25
and gout, 25
and joint pressure, 19, 25
and progressive daytime fatigue,
24–25
and sleep problems, 24–25
weight lifting. *See* weight training
weight loss
and alcohol use, 115
alternative treatments, 119–120
benefits, 126
calories and, 48–51
carbohydrate restriction and, 125
cathartics, 39
change of environment and, 35
discipline and, 4, 33, 34
diuretics, 39
eggs and, 118
exercise and. *See* exercise
fats and, 81–82
goals, realistic, 4
liquid meal replacements, 99
medications, 120
motivation and, 4, 18, 33
nuts and, 89
patience and, 33, 34
quick fix, 1, 37
sauna, 39
speed of, 39–40
weight training and, 48–51
weight training
benefits for elderly, 50–51
cautions for, 49
sample program, 50*t*
Weight Watchers, 54
weight-loss programs, meal
frequency, 54

Western diet, and obesity, 12
white chardonnay, source of
flavonoids, 110
whole grain products
benefits for thin people, 66–67
low glycemic index/load and, 65
positive effects on diabetes risk,
66
positive effects on stroke risk, 65,
66
Wife's Salad (recipe), 129
wine
benefits, 110
protective effects of, 114
source of flavonoids, 109
wine-only diet, 1
women
and alcohol intake, 113
and breast cancer. *See* breast
cancer
calories burned exercising, 42
cardio-metabolic syndrome
factors, 29
effects of obesity on hormonal
and reproductive system, 26
exercise rate, 51
obesity rate, 12
pregnant, and omega-3s, 86
premature deaths, 26
and uterine cancer, 24
work, as exercise, 14

Z

Zone diet, 67
Zucchini and Yellow Summer
Squash (recipe), 129